FAST FACTS

Disorders of the Hair and Scalp

Indispensable

Guides to

Clinical

Practice

Anne Farrell
Consultant Dermatologist,
Kent and Sussex Hospital,
Tunbridge Wells, UK

Rodney Sinclair
Consultant Dermatologist,
St Vincent Hospital,
Melbourne, Australia

Rodney Dawber
Consultant Dermatologist,
The Oxford Radcliffe Hospital,
Oxford, UK

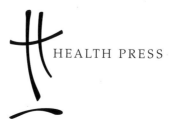

HEALTH PRESS

Oxford

Fast Facts – Disorders of the Hair and Scalp
First published 2000

Text © 2000 Anne Farrell, Rodney Sinclair, Rodney Dawber
© 2000 in this edition Health Press Limited
Elizabeth House, Queen Street, Abingdon, Oxford OX14 3JR, UK

Tel: +44 (0)1235 523233
Fax: +44 (0)1235 523238

Fast Facts is a trade mark of Health Press Limited.

The publisher and the authors have made every effort to ensure the
accuracy of this book, but cannot accept responsibility for any errors
or omissions.

A CIP catalogue record for this title is available from the British Library.

ISBN 1-899541-03-9

Farrell, A. (Anne)
Fast Facts – Disorders of the Hair and Scalp/
Anne Farrell, Rodney Sinclair, Rodney Dawber

Illustrated by Dee McLean, London, UK.

Printed by Fine Print (Services) Ltd, Oxford, UK.

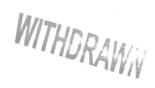

Glossary

5α-dihydrotestosterone: an androgen converted from testosterone by the action of 5α-reductase

5α-reductase: an enzyme catalysing the conversion of testosterone to 5α-dihydrotestosterone

Alopecia: baldness

Alopecia areata: an autoimmune condition resulting in patchy baldness and exclamation-mark hairs

Alopecia totalis: alopecia areata resulting in complete loss of scalp hair

Anagen: the growth phase of the hair cycle

Arrector pili: involuntary muscles attached to the hair follicles – on contraction, the hairs become erect

Atrichia congenita: a condition resulting in total and permanent absence of scalp hair

Bulla: a large and watery blister

Catagen: the involution (shrinkage) phase of the hair cycle

Cuticle: the outermost part of the hair shaft, comprising between 5 and 10 overlapping cell layers

Ectothrix: a fungal infection in which spores are generated on the hair shaft

Endothrix: a fungal infection in which spores are generated within the cortex of the hair

Exclamation-mark hair: seen in alopecia areata, hair that tapers and is narrowest close to the scalp

FSH: follicle-stimulating hormone, secreted by the anterior pituitary gland

Hair cycle: the repetitive sequence of growth and rest undergone by each hair follicle

Hypertrichosis: excessive hairiness at unusual sites

Ichthyosis: dry and scaly skin

Imbricated: with overlapping edges

Keratin: a structural protein

Kerion: a painful inflammatory abscess-like mass resulting from ringworm infection

Lanugo: soft downy hair that covers a fetus, occasionally seen on neonates, particularly if premature

LE: lupus erythematosus, an autoimmune disease

LH: luteinizing hormone, secreted by the anterior pituitary gland

Marie Unna syndrome: an autosomal dominant disorder in which hair becomes coarse and twisted and is progressively lost from the scalp as the hair follicles are destroyed by scarring

Melanization: the process of imparting the dark pigment melanin

Monilethrix: a rare, inherited defect of the hair follicle characterized by beaded hairs that break easily

Morphoea: localized scleroderma

Netherton's syndrome: a hereditary condition in which an ichthyosiform erythroderma called ichthyosis linearis circumflexa is combined with fragile hair with invaginate nodes (trichorrhexis invaginata)

Pili torti: the presence of fragile hairs that are flattened and twisted through 180° at irregular intervals along the shaft

Progeria: a genetic disorder characterized by premature ageing

Scutula: a yellowish, cup-shaped crust seen in tinea capitis, which is caused by *Trichophyton schoenleinii*

SHBG: sex hormone-binding globulin, a protein that binds circulating testosterone

Spangled hair: appearance of twisted hair that reflects the light at various angles; hair with alternating light and dark bands also has this appearance

Telogen: the resting phase of the hair cycle

Terminal hair: hair that is longer and coarser than vellus hair

Tinea capitis: ringworm of the scalp in which the basic feature is invasion of hair shafts by a dermatophyte fungus

Trichotillomania: artefactual damage resulting from hair pulling

Uncombable hair: an autosomal, dominantly inherited genodermatosis, characterized by triangular hairs

Vellus hair: the short, downy hair that replaces lanugo before or shortly after birth on hair-bearing skin apart from the scalp

Weathering: the process that results in hair becoming jagged and progressively breaking off, caused by chemical and physical insults

Introduction

Warm-blooded mammals owe much of their evolutionary success to the insulation provided by their hairy covering. Paradoxically, the movement of humans from their ancestral forest home to populate the globe was linked with a reversion to relative nudity. Among mammals, hair serves many purposes. In particular, it is concerned with sexual and social communication, for example, the mane of the lion, the beard of the human male or the magnificent display of scalp hair paraded by many humans, albeit with cosmetic assistance. It also plays a role in assisting the dispersal of scents secreted by adjacent sebaceous or apocrine glands.

Although, in humans, none of the functions of hair is vital, its psychological importance is immense and diseases resulting in cosmetic alterations can be a source of significant psychological distress. The aim of this book is to deal with hair problems as they usually present in clinical practice. We hope that this book will provide healthcare workers with a practical guide to diagnose and manage these conditions effectively, and so bring comfort to the thousands of individuals with hair and scalp disorders.

CHAPTER 1
Anatomy and physiology

Embryology

The sequence of events by which the hair follicle is formed in the fetus is partly recapitulated in each adult cycle. The first sign of hair development occurs between about 9 and 12 weeks of gestational age. Crowding of cells in the basal layer of the fetal epidermis is associated with aggregation of mesenchymal cells just below it (Figure 1.1).

The epidermal cells grow downwards to form a solid column of cells called the 'hair peg', the broad tip of which becomes slightly concave. It carries before it the aggregation of mesenchymal cells, which will form the dermal papilla and dermal sheath. As the hair peg grows down, the

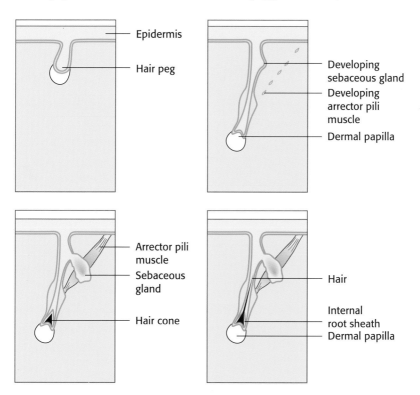

Figure 1.1 The embryological development of hair.

9

advancing extremity becomes bulbous ('the hair bulb' or 'bulbous hair peg') and the cavity at the tip deepens to enclose the dermal papilla. The rapidly dividing cells in the bulb surrounding the dermal papilla make up the hair matrix. Two swellings then appear – the upper swelling is the precursor of the sebaceous gland, the lower (the bulge or Wulst) will be the site of attachment of the arrector pili muscle. In many follicles, a third bulb appears above the sebaceous gland bud – in some areas of the skin, notably the axilla, groin, genital skin, areola and face, this will form the apocrine gland, while elsewhere it involutes.

Above the hair matrix, a cone of cells differentiates to form hair, organizing into the cuticle and cortex. A second concentric cone differentiates around it to form the inner root sheath. Three components of the inner root sheath develop – the outer of these is Henle's layer, inside this is Huxley's layer and then inside this is the cuticle of the inner root sheath. The invaginated epidermis forms the outer root sheath and surrounding this is a connective tissue layer. These developmental events depend on a complex series of interactive messages between the dermis and epidermis.

The first hair follicles start to appear in the regions of the eyebrows, upper lip and chin at about 9 weeks of embryonic development. Hair follicle development proceeds in a cephalocaudal direction and is complete by 22 weeks. This first coat of fine lanugo hair is shed *in utero* about 1 month before birth. The second coat of lanugo, covering all areas except the scalp where there is longer hair of thicker calibre, is lost almost imperceptibly during the first 3–4 months of life. These first two coats are synchronized in growth and in sequence of shedding. Thereafter, an unsynchronized (or mosaic) pattern of growth occurs.

As the body surface increases, there is a decrease in actual density of follicles. It is generally accepted that, under normal circumstances, new follicles cannot develop in adult skin. The total is estimated to be 5 million, of which about 1 million are on the head and perhaps 100 000 in the scalp. There appear to be no significant sexual or racial differences in follicle number.

Anatomy

The structure of the adult hair follicle is shown in Figure 1.2. As described above, the outer root sheath derives from the epidermis and structures inside this arise from the hair matrix in the bulb. Active cell division occurs in the bulb from where cells stream upwards and undergo the successive phases of orientation into layers, hardening and keratinization.

As the cortical cells of the hair move upwards, they produce increasing amounts of cytoplasmic microfibrils parallel to the long axes of both the cell and the hair follicle. These are composed of keratins, which are a group of insoluble cysteine-containing helical protein complexes. The microfibrils become aggregated into macrofibrils of 0.1–0.4 µm in diameter. As the cells move up the hair follicle, many of the cellular organelles are lost. Eventually the cell nucleus is lost, leaving fully keratinized 'dead' cortical cells, approximately 3–6 µm in diameter and up to 100 µm long, which retain a membranous nuclear outline (nuclear 'ghost'). By this stage, a dense amorphous matrix has formed, composed of sulphur-rich proteins with many cysteine links within which the macrofibrils are orientated longitudinally.

The cuticle consists of five to ten overlapping cell layers, each 350–450 nm thick. From the outside, the scales appear to be imbricated, overlapping like the tiles on a roof (Figure 1.3). The scale margins are intact over the newly formed part of the hair, but as the hair emerges from the skin the margins become jagged and progressively break off ('weathering'). The 'environmental' outer surface of each cuticular cell has a very clear A-layer, which is rich in high-sulphur protein; this protects the cuticular cells from premature breakdown due to chemical and physical insults.

Each of the three layers of the inner root sheath undergoes keratinization and though the rates of maturation are different, the patterns of change are identical. This involves the development of keratin filaments and trichohyaline granules within the cytoplasm. The inner root sheath hardens before the presumptive hair within it, and it is consequently thought to control the definitive shape of the hair shaft in health and in many genetic diseases that result in abnormal hair morphology.

At the level of the follicular canal, desmosomes (which mediate adhesion between the cells of the outer root sheath) break down, and the outer root sheath cells are shed into the follicular canal, singly or in groups.

Pigmentation of hair is caused by functional melanocytes present among cells of the hair matrix in the bulb at the apex of the dermal papilla. These melanocytes donate melanosomes, which contain the pigment

11

(a)

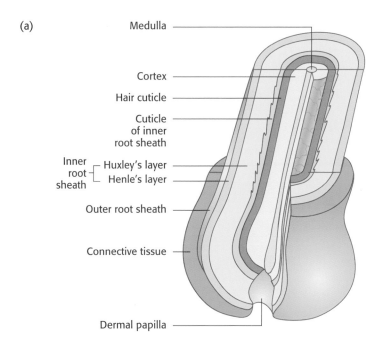

Medulla

Cortex

Hair cuticle

Cuticle of inner root sheath

Inner root sheath {
 Huxley's layer
 Henle's layer

Outer root sheath

Connective tissue

Dermal papilla

(b)

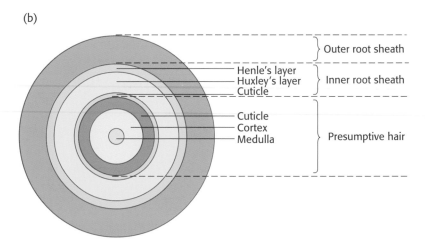

Outer root sheath

Henle's layer
Huxley's layer
Cuticle

Inner root sheath

Cuticle
Cortex
Medulla

Presumptive hair

Figure 1.2 The hair follicle: (a) section through a hair follicle; (b) cross-section of a follicle; (c) histology of the hair follicle (haematoxylin and eosin staining); (d) longitudinal section through a hair shaft at the root end.

(c)

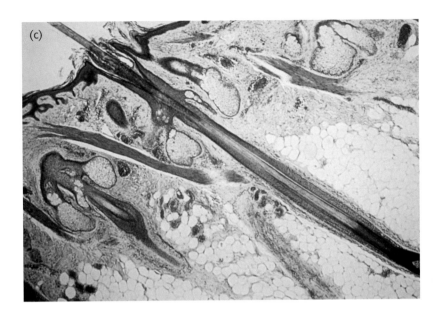

(d)

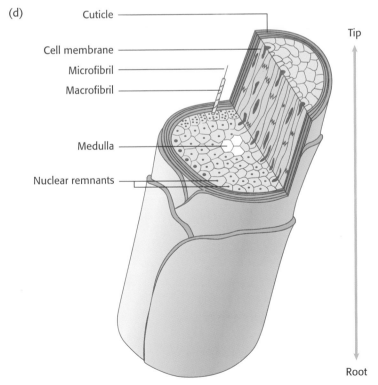

Cuticle

Cell membrane

Microfibril

Macrofibril

Medulla

Nuclear remnants

Tip

Root

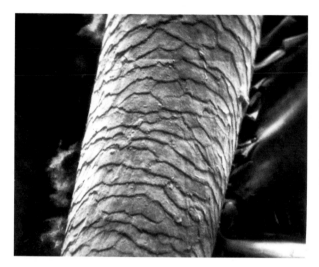

Figure 1.3
Scanning electron microscopy of hair showing the overlapping keratin-rich cells on the cuticle surface.

melanin, to the hair matrix cells that will eventually differentiate to form the hair cortex. No pigment is donated to the cuticular cells or internal root sheath.

An additional feature of some terminal, but not vellus or lanugo, hairs is the presence of medullary cells in the centres of the follicles. These develop vacuoles at the level of the epidermis, some of which become air-filled, forming an interrupted air-filled core in the centre of the hair (the medulla).

The hair cycle

From the time of its formation, each hair follicle undergoes a repetitive sequence of growth and rest known as the 'hair cycle'. The growth phase is called 'anagen' and it is followed by an involution phase ('catagen') and then by a resting phase ('telogen') (Figures 1.4 and 1.5). The relative duration of each phase of the cycle varies with the age of the individual and the region of the body and can be modified by a variety of factors, local and systemic.

Anagen. The sequence of events in anagen recapitulates those occurring during fetal development, to an extent. In the first stage of anagen, cells at the base of the epithelial sac (the secondary germ) begin to show mitotic activity. In stage 2, they start to grow down to enclose the dermal papilla. At the same time, the inner root sheath appears as a keratinized plate-like

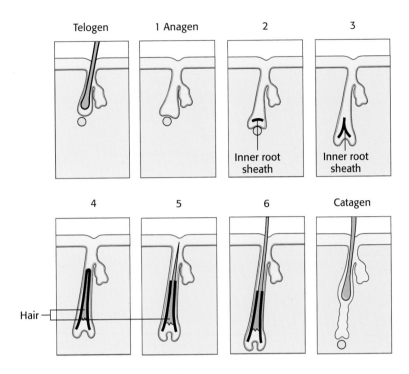

Figure 1.4 The stages of the hair cycle.

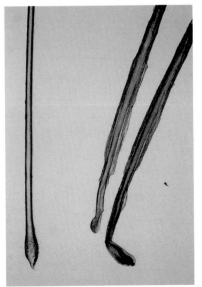

Figure 1.5 A photomicrograph of three hair shafts. The left shaft has the characteristic 'drumstick' appearance of a telogen bulb. The middle shaft has a tapered straight bulb surrounded by a loose atrophic sack and is a catagen bulb. The shaft on the right has a densely pigmented and distorted bulb with an extravagant collar of external root sheath and is typical of an anagen bulb.

structure overlying the matrix. As the follicle enters anagen 3, the keratinizing inner root sheath starts to form a conical shape beneath which the cortex starts to differentiate. Melanogenesis also starts within the matrix. In anagen 4, the cortex is keratinizing but has not yet penetrated the inner root sheath; pigment donation to the cortical cells is evident. In anagen 5, the developing hair shaft finally penetrates the inner root sheath at the level of the sebaceous duct. Anagen 6 represents the fully developed follicle. Stages 1–5 are sometimes collectively known as 'pro-anagen', and stage 6 is known as 'met-anagen'.

The duration of anagen varies greatly between species, regionally within the same species, with season and with age. In human vellus follicles of both sexes, the periods of activity range from about 40 to 80 days. Estimated averages of 54 and 28 days have been made for the thighs and arms, respectively, of Caucasoid males, and 22 days for each of these sites in females. In the human scalp, anagen may last for 3–7 years.

Catagen. Towards the end of anagen, mitosis in the matrix decreases and then stops. The follicle then enters catagen. The middle region of the bulb becomes constricted, but distal to this constriction the expanded base of the hair continues to keratinize and becomes club-shaped. Melanization ceases just before entry into catagen, so the club remains non-pigmented. The lower portion of the outer root sheath undergoes apoptotic degeneration and the base of the follicle, together with the club hair, moves upwards to eventually lie at the level of the arrector insertion. The space that is left below is filled with undifferentiated cells forming an elongated column. The inner root sheath disintegrates and disappears. The hair club is held in place by a capsule of epithelial cells, attached by keratinized fibres. The outer root sheath thickens, particularly its basement membrane (often referred to as the 'glassy' or 'vitreous' membrane). The dermal papilla remains closely associated with the base of the follicle. Catagen lasts approximately 2 weeks in the human scalp.

Telogen. This is the resting phase of the hair cycle. The club is held in the epithelial sac and may be retained until the next anagen is well advanced. The dermal papilla, still closely associated with the base of the follicular epithelium, has lost its blood supply during catagen and now appears as a tightly packed ball of cells. When the next cell cycle starts, the secondary germ forms, probably from the stem cell bulge area adjacent to the arrector pili insert, and anagen commences. The old club hair is shed once all its cell attachments are lost.

At any one time, approximately 13% of the follicles in the human scalp are in telogen, though the range is large (it has been recorded as 4–24%). Only 1% or fewer are in catagen. If there are about 100 000 follicles in the scalp and their period is about 1000 days, about 100 hairs ought to be lost each day. In practice, the average recovery of shed hairs is usually rather lower, and over 100 is regarded as high. Follicles throughout the body, as well as those on the scalp, are out of synchrony and, indeed, have different periodicities. Each hair follicle appears to have an intrinsic rhythm. Plucking of hairs from resting follicles brings forward the next period of activity, and such follicles continue out of phase with their neighbours, at least for a time. The nature of the intrinsic control of the hair cycle and the mechanism by which epilation or wounding affect it are unknown. One hypothesis is that a mitotic inhibitor accumulates during anagen and is gradually used up or dispersed during telogen. Another is that growth-promoting wound hormones are released by epilation.

Hair types

Different types of hair may be produced by different kinds of follicle, and the type of hair produced in any particular follicle can change with age or under the influence of hormones. Prenatal lanugo may be retained throughout life in the rare hereditary syndrome hypertrichosis lanuginosa. Postnatal hair may be divided at the two extremes into two kinds:

- vellus hair, which is soft, unmedullated, occasionally pigmented and seldom more than 2 cm long
- terminal hair, which is longer, coarser, and often medullated and pigmented.
  However, there is a range of intermediate kinds. Before puberty, terminal hair is normally limited to the scalp, eyebrows and eyelashes. After puberty, secondary sexual 'terminal' hair develops from vellus hair in response to androgens.

Human vellus hairs act as very sensitive and subtle tactile nerve endings, and other hair fibres are important in specific conditioned reactions – nostril hairs in sneezing and eyelashes in blinking, for example.

Hormonal influences on the hair cycle

Irrespective of intrinsic control, the overall timing of the cyclic events also appears to be influenced by systemic factors. This systemic control may embody components as yet unknown.

Human hair is profoundly affected by the level of unbound thyroid hormones. In some studies, up to 10% of those who complained of hair loss were diagnosed as suffering from hypothyroidism. Mean hair diameter in these subjects was reduced. The proportion of roots in telogen has been shown to be abnormally high in hairs plucked from the occipital and parietal areas of hypothyroid subjects; treatment with thyroid hormone restored it to normal after 8 weeks.

The phenomenon of postpartum hair loss also appears to result from a hormonally mediated change in the cycles of scalp follicles. A loss of hairs at about two to three times the normal rate gives rise to a transient alopecia about 4–6 months after delivery. At this time, the proportion of hairs in telogen can be as high as 50%, in contrast with late pregnancy, when it may be less than 5%.

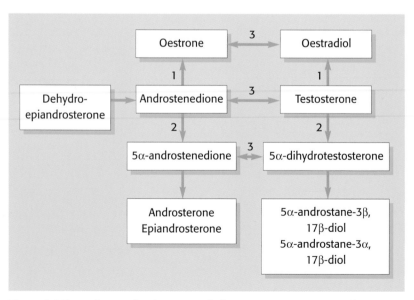

Figure 1.6 The pathways of androgen metabolism. 1, Aromatase; 2, 5α-reductase; 3, 17β-hydroxysteroid dehydrogenase.

Influence of androgens on hair growth. In addition to exerting influence on the timing of the follicular cycle, androgens are particularly important in determining the pattern of adult hair growth. The growth of facial, trunk and extremity hair in the male, and of pubic and axillary hair in both sexes, is clearly dependent on androgens. The development of such hair at and after puberty is, in broad terms, and at least initially, in parallel with the rise in levels of androgens from testicular, adrenocortical and ovarian sources. The rise occurs in both sexes, but is somewhat steeper in boys than in girls.

Body hair. Direct evidence of the role of testicular androgen is provided by the fact that castration reduces growth of the human beard, whereas testosterone stimulates it in eunuchs and old men. Since very obvious facial and body hair is normally absent from women, growth appears to require high levels of the hormone and, since it is usually deficient in men with 5α-reductase deficiency, it seems that metabolism of testosterone to 5α-dihydrotestosterone is mandatory. The pathways of androgen metabolism are shown in Figure 1.6. The role of androgen is further demonstrated in the treatment of hirsute women with the anti-androgen cyproterone acetate, which reduces the definitive length, rate of growth, diameter and extent of medullation of the thigh hairs. Although cyproterone acetate does lower plasma androgen levels, its main mode of action appears to be via competition for the androgen receptors in the hair follicle.

Growth of pubic and axillary hair is undoubtedly androgen dependent, as is that on the backs of hands, finger, pinna and the tip of the nose. This hair is deficient in testicular feminization (a condition in which genetic males develop as females because of a lack of intracellular androgen receptors), and in women suffering from adrenal insufficiency. However, it is present in the condition type II incomplete hermaphroditism, in which genetic males lack 5α-reductase even though their plasma testosterone is normal. Therefore, it seems that growth of the pubic hair does not require the formation of dihydrotestosterone.

Scalp hair differs in that its growth does not require any androgenic stimulus. However, in genetically predisposed subjects, androgen is paradoxically responsible for postpubertal hair miniaturization on the vertex of the scalp. The existence of testosterone receptors in scalp hair follicles is implied by the fact that in females, androgenetic alopecia can be alleviated by oral anti-androgens. Not only are androgen receptors present, as demonstrated by studies of scalp biopsy specimens, but the scalp hair follicles also have active androgen metabolism as has been directly demonstrated in cultured dermal papilla cells. The additional necessity for 5α-reductase is suggested by evidence that the male bald scalp has a greater capacity than the non-bald scalp to convert testosterone to dihydrotestosterone and that recession of the frontal hairline does not occur in cases of familial male pseudo-hermaphroditism involving 5α-reductase deficiency.

Male-pattern baldness. The question as to whether male-pattern baldness is associated with other signs of virility or abnormal androgen levels has been debated. Evidence that it is correlated with hairiness of the chest appears to be contradicted by a failure to find any association with density of body hair, skin and muscle thickness, or rate of sebum excretion. However, the occasional finding that, despite normal plasma testosterone, bald men tend to have lower sex hormone-binding globulin (SHBG) and higher salivary testosterone does suggest that they might have higher levels of available androgen.

Growth-hormone deficiency. The findings that growth-hormone-deficient children are less responsive to androgens than non-deficient children, and that growth hormone is a synergistic factor necessary for fully effective testosterone, with respect to protein anabolism, growth promotion and androgenicity, imply that hypophysial hormones also play a significant role.

Racial and individual variation

Wide, genetically determined variations in the pattern and amount of hair growth can be observed between races and between individuals. The most striking differences are seen in scalp hair. It is a common observation that Mongoloids tend to have straight hair, Negroids curly hair and Caucasoids a range of textures and curl. According to several authors, the macroscopic appearance of hair is related to its cross-section. Thus Mongoloid hair is the widest and is circular, Negroid hair is oval, and Caucasoid hair is moderately elliptical and finer than Mongoloid. Other evidence suggests that the shape of the follicle determines hair form: the Negroid follicle is helical, the Mongoloid completely straight, and the Caucasoid varies between these extremes. However, even a straight Caucasoid follicle may produce a hair with an oval cross section. Significant variations between populations can be shown for a number of other measurements such as medullation, cuticular scale count, kinking and average curvature.

Mongoloids, both male and female, have less pubic, axillary, beard and body hair than Caucasoids. The surface area covered by coarse beard hairs and the weight of hairs grown per day are lower in Japanese than in Caucasians, as are the mean number of axillary hairs and their daily growth rate.

The growth of coarse hairs on the rim of the helix (hypertrichosis of the pinna) occurs between the ages of 17 and 45 years in many males, being particularly obvious among the Bengali and Sinhalese. The character is well known to geneticists as a possible example of Y-linked inheritance. In other races, few or many coarse hairs may grow on the helix or on other regions of the pinna, usually after the third decade. The patterns have been classified but their modes of inheritance are unknown.

Seasonal changes

Clear and statistically significant data on seasonal variation have been provided by several studies of young adults in Europe. Hair loss reached a peak around August or September, when the fewest follicles were in anagen. At this time, the average loss of hairs was about 60 per day, more than double that seen in March and compatible with the observed increase from 10% to 20% in the proportion of follicles in telogen. However, the diameter of growing scalp hairs exhibited no significant seasonal fluctuations.

The rate of beard growth showed very significant seasonal variation. It was lowest in January and February, and from March it increased steadily to reach a peak in July.

CHAPTER 2
Diffuse hair loss

Diffuse hair loss occurring in the absence of scalp inflammation is usually a matter of great concern for those affected, particularly women, who do not generally expect to experience hair thinning. The most frequent cause in the western world is androgenetic alopecia (common baldness/male-pattern alopecia/pattern baldness), but other causes include:

- telogen effluvium
- thyroid disease
- iron deficiency
- protein deficiency.

Any of these can exacerbate androgenetic alopecia.

In men, androgenetic alopecia causes the typical temporal recession (thinning of the hair around the temples) and thinning of the vertex (well described by Hamilton and later by Norwood) (Figure 2.1), while in women, the pattern is a more diffuse alopecia (as described by Ludwig) (Figure 2.2).

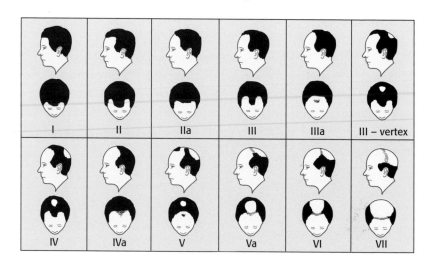

Figure 2.1 Hamilton and Norwood patterns of common baldness as seen in men. Adapted from Norwood OT and Schiell RD, *Hair Transplant Surgery*. 2nd edition, 1984. Courtesy of Charles C Thomas, Publisher Ltd., Springfield, Illinois, USA.

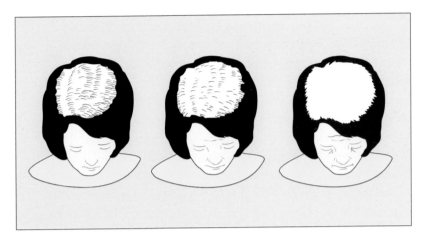

Figure 2.2 Common pattern baldness as seen in women (as described by Ludwig).

Because hair loss is more widely accepted as the natural maturation of the male scalp, it is less often a cause for a medical consultation in men, though with the increasing pressure to 'look young', more men are now seeking advice about hair loss. When assessing diffuse hair loss, it is important to examine the scalp closely to exclude an inflammatory scalp disorder or a scarring alopecia (see Chapter 4).

Androgenetic alopecia

Common baldness is a genetically determined physiological event that occurs during the lifetime of most men and women, though the exact mode of inheritance is not known. The physiological change involves a shortening of the anagen phase of the hair cycle and a consequent increase in the proportion of telogen hairs. Linear growth is only minimally reduced. Structurally, the terminal hair follicles progressively transform into small 'vellus' follicles, but these differ from true vellus follicles by still retaining some remnants of the arrector pili muscles (i.e. a 'miniaturization' process occurs). Scalp biopsies show that early on in the process there is also a mild degree of perifollicular inflammation, which results in destruction of the connective tissue sheath, the remains of which can be seen as 'streamers'. Reduced blood flow to the region of scalp involved has also been demonstrated, but whether this precedes or follows the baldness is unknown.

23

Genetic basis. Some studies have suggested an autosomal dominant inheritance with increased penetrance in the male, while others have supported a multifactorial inheritance. It is as yet unclear whether the patterns of inheritance differ between early- (before the age of 30 years) and late-onset baldness. It is anticipated that gene-linkage studies will identify genes involved in the inheritance of androgenetic alopecia.

Disturbance in sebaceous activity. Early theories that a disturbance in sebaceous activity is a cause of common baldness have not been substantiated. Studies have failed to show a difference between the rate of production of sebum in bald men and those with a full head of hair. No qualitative differences have been found in the skin surface lipids.

Androgens. The role of androgens and their interaction with genetic factors were demonstrated by Hamilton. He reported that baldness did not occur in 10 eunuchoids, 10 men castrated at puberty and 34 men castrated during adolescence, but that administration of testosterone led to baldness in those who were genetically predisposed. On discontinuing testosterone, the baldness did not progress though it did not reverse. Furthermore, males suffering from syndromes of androgen insensitivity, such as 5α-reductase deficiency, fail to develop temporal recession after puberty. However, a number of studies involving men have failed to show a correlation between testosterone levels and baldness. In women, on the other hand, the degree of baldness can be associated with elevated levels of circulating androgens; changes in hair pattern most frequently occur after the menopause when a more 'androgenetic' environment occurs. A number of women presenting with androgenetic alopecia have polycystic ovary syndrome. Nevertheless, many women who develop androgenetic alopecia have normal levels of circulating androgens, and there are some women who do not develop baldness despite having significantly abnormal levels of androgens, though they do become hirsute. It appears that the essential inherited factor responsible for androgenetic alopecia is the manner in which the follicles of the frontal and vertex regions of the scalp react to androgens. It is well established that the pilo-sebaceous unit can metabolize a wide range of androgens. More recently, androgen receptors have been demonstrated in the dermal papilla.

Assessment of women with androgenetic alopecia includes:

- enquiring about amenorrhoea or oligomenorrhoea which, if present, may suggest polycystic ovary disease
- enquiring about galactorrhoea, as elevated prolactin levels can result in androgenetic alopecia by displacing testosterone from SHBG
- examination for hirsutism and evidence of virilization.

Baseline investigations should include assessment of the levels of:

- prolactin
- luteinizing hormone (LH)
- follicle-stimulating hormone (FSH)
- testosterone
- SHBG.

It is also useful to check that there are no abnormalities in thyroid function, and iron and ferritin levels, which might exacerbate androgenetic alopecia.

Treatment. The only topical preparation that has, to date, been demonstrated to show some effectiveness in androgenetic alopecia is minoxidil. This piperidinopyrimidine derivative is a potent vasodilator that was originally used in the treatment of hypertension. Several studies have reported that when it is applied topically, twice daily, as a 2% solution, it results in the conversion of some vellus-like hairs to terminal hairs and results in moderate to dense regrowth of hair in 24–59% of individuals. However, a uniform covering of the bald areas is seen in fewer than 10% of subjects, and at least in men, those patients who respond best are younger, have a smaller area of hair loss and are in the early stages of balding. Additional benefit has recently been shown using the 5% minoxidil solution.

The mode of action of minoxidil is uncertain – it does not have anti-androgenic properties and an increase in cutaneous blood flow has not been clearly demonstrated. Topical minoxidil appears to be well tolerated. The main side-effect is occasional local irritation and contact dermatitis (low incidence). The benefits only last for as long as the topical minoxidil is applied; on discontinuing the applications, hair loss recurs 3–6 months later, and reaches the level that it would have reached had the minoxidil not been used.

Other therapeutic measures reported to lead to some improvement in individual cases include drugs with anti-androgenic properties, such as cyproterone acetate, spironolactone, cimetidine, ketoconazole and flutamide, but reports of their efficacy are 'uncontrolled'. Because of their anti-androgenic properties, these drugs have been used predominantly in females, though when cyproterone acetate was used to treat persistent male sex offenders, androgenetic alopecia in these men was said to improve.

Of these drugs, only cyproterone acetate has been studied extensively, though even these studies concentrated on its effect on hirsutism, and its effects on scalp hair were reported as incidental findings. Daily doses of 50–100 mg may prevent further progression of hair loss, though there is little evidence to support its use to encourage hair regrowth. Cyproterone acetate at a dose of 2 mg combined with ethinyloestradiol (Dianette®, Schering Healthcare) may maintain the improvement gained. However, there are no long-term prospective trials of its use in androgenetic alopecia. Side-effects include lassitude, weight gain, breast tenderness, loss of libido and nausea; because it has the potential to feminize a male fetus, it should be used in conjunction with adequate contraception in premenopausal women. There has also been concern about the hepatic effects of cyproterone acetate: fulminant hepatitis has been reported, but the majority of cases were in men receiving a high dose for prostate cancer. It is therefore advisable to stop cyproterone acetate in a patient who develops signs of hepatotoxicity. There have also been a handful of reports of hepatocellular cancer occurring in patients who were receiving cyproterone acetate, but again these have been associated with high doses. There are no epidemiological data linking the drug with development of liver tumours.

A subjective improvement in androgenetic alopecia has been reported with oral spironolactone, although patients also complained of mood swings, irregular menses and breast tenderness. Flutamide is a pure anti-androgen, mainly studied in hirsutism, but there are anecdotal reports of its effectiveness in androgenetic alopecia. It has also been reported to be potentially hepatotoxic and regular monitoring of liver function is recommended. It is not recommended in any but the most recalcitrant cases.

A recent promising development for the treatment of androgenetic alopecia is finasteride. This is a selective inhibitor of the type 2 isoenzyme of 5α-reductase, which converts testosterone to dihydrotestosterone (DHT). The type 1 isoenzyme is found predominantly in the skin, located in sebaceous glands, epidermal and follicular keratinocytes, dermal papilla cells, sweat glands and fibroblasts. Type 2 is found in the liver, prostate, epididymis, seminal vesicles, and inner root sheath of the hair follicle. Both forms of 5α-reductase isoenzyme are present in frontal hair follicles of women and men with androgenetic alopecia, and lower levels are also present in occipital hair follicles (which are more 'androgen resistant'). Patients with 5α-reductase deficiency do not develop androgenetic alopecia, and elevated levels of DHT have been observed in the hair follicles of scalps of patients with androgenetic alopecia. This has led to trials of finasteride in men with common baldness which have reported it to be beneficial. In detailed human studies, finasteride, 1 mg/day orally, resulted in decreases in the level of DHT in the scalp and serum compared with placebo, with no clinically important changes in serum LH, FSH or testosterone. Safety and tolerability profiles are excellent and, at a dose of 1 mg/day, there are no significant adverse effects and no statistically significant impairment of male fertility compared with placebo. However, because of its potential feminizing effect on the male fetus, it is contraindicated in women who are or may become pregnant. Furthermore, these women should not handle crushed or broken tablets.

Although a number of drugs (including diazoxide, minoxidil, viprostol, benoxaprofen and cyclosporin A), when given systemically, have been reported to lead to an improvement in androgenetic alopecia as part of a general hypertrichosis, because of their side-effect profiles they are not recommended for androgenetic alopecia.

Telogen effluvium

As part of the natural hair growth cycle, hairs in the telogen phase are shed from all areas of the scalp on a daily basis. Normally, these follicles then re-enter anagen so that no obvious hair thinning is apparent. However, if a large number of hair follicles enter catagen together, diffuse excessive hair loss is observed 2–3 months later. Such a pattern may be seen following significant physical or emotional stress (Table 2.1). However the precise mechanism causing the sudden diffuse shedding of telogen hair is not known. If the physical or emotional stress passes, the hair usually regrows.

27

TABLE 2.1

Causes of diffuse, excessive hair loss

- Childbirth
- High fever
- Haemorrhage
- Sudden starvation
- Malignancy
- Significant surgery
- Severe impairment of liver or renal function
- Severe emotional stress
- Certain drugs
- Industrial or accidental exposure to certain chemicals

Other causes of diffuse hair loss

Sometimes slow onset of hair thinning is seen in the absence of obvious hair shedding if hairs at the end of a normal telogen fail to re-enter anagen. This is the pattern more often seen in iron-deficiency anaemia, hypothyroidism and hypopituitarism.

Iron deficiency may still be present despite normal full blood count and some authors maintain that iron storage deficiency sufficient to cause hair loss may still be present even with normal serum iron levels if the serum ferritin is low.

Hypothyroidism. Diffuse hair loss occurring in hypothyroidism is theoretically reversible on administering thyroxine, but if the hypothyroidism has been present over a long time period, it can result in permanent miniaturization of the hair follicles.

Pregnancy. Diffuse hair thinning commonly occurs after pregnancy (see Chapter 1). Full recovery is usually by 4–9 months, assuming adequate diet.

Oral contraceptive pill. There has been debate over whether the oral contraceptive pill causes hair loss but few detailed studies have been performed. Whether a particular oral contraceptive pill is likely to cause hair loss seems to depend on whether it has a net androgenic effect. The observation that diffuse hair loss occurs on discontinuing the oral contraceptive has been better documented and the mechanism is probably similar to, but usually less dramatic than, that causing hair loss following pregnancy.

Inadequate diet. Protein-calorie malnutrition, essential fatty acid deficiency or zinc deficiency due to inadequate diet or inadequate supplementation in parenteral nutrition can also result in diffuse hair loss. It improves when the nutritional deficiencies are corrected.

Secondary syphilis. Diffuse hair loss can be a feature of secondary syphilis, but here the hair typically has a 'moth-eaten' appearance and tends to regrow after 4–6 months.

Chronic renal failure can also result in diffuse hair loss, but by a mechanism that is poorly understood at present; this hair loss is not reversed following dialysis.

Certain drugs can cause hair loss (Table 2.2); some induce shedding of anagen hair and/or premature catagen followed by telogen shedding, while

---

TABLE 2.2

Some drugs and other substances that can cause hair loss

• Allopurinol	• Doxorubicin
• β-blockers	• Heparin
• Borax	• Lithium
• Bromocriptine	• Mercury
• Carbamazepine	• Pitressin
• Clofibrate	• Retinoids
• Colchicine	• Sodium valproate
• Coumarins	• Thallium
• Cyclophosphamide	• Triparanol

with other substances, the precise mechanism underlying hair loss is not established.

Chemical agents. Repeated damage to hair shafts by chemical agents used for cosmetic purposes, such as hair dyes, bleaches and perm solutions, should also be remembered as possible causes; a clue is weathering of the hair shaft seen on light microscopy.

Assessment

Assessment of patients with diffuse hair loss should include:

- detailed medical history
- full blood count
- serum iron and ferritin measurement
- liver, renal and thyroid function tests
- microscopy of hair (to look for evidence of weathering, fractured hairs of cytotoxic injury or any congenital shaft abnormalities that may have made the hair shaft more susceptible to trauma).

CHAPTER 3

Patchy hair loss

The two most common causes of patchy hair loss are alopecia areata and trichotillomania (artefactual damage as a result of hair pulling).

Alopecia areata

The characteristic presentation of alopecia areata is the appearance of a well-circumscribed, totally bald, smooth patch, often with the presence of exclamation-mark hairs at the border (Figures 3.1–3.3). In the majority of cases, the lesion is asymptomatic and may be noticed by the patient only by chance, though some patients do complain of local irritation or paraesthesia preceding the hair loss. The reason why white hairs appear to be relatively spared compared with pigmented hairs is poorly understood, but this phenomenon may be the explanation behind reports of 'hair turning white overnight' in historical figures such as Marie Antoinette.

It has been claimed that the scalp is the first site to be affected in 60% of cases but all sites of the body may be involved. The subsequent progress is varied; the initial patch of hair loss may regrow within a few months, though new hair is often white and finer than hair elsewhere. Alternatively new areas of hair loss may develop in some cases, resulting in total hair loss (Figure 3.4). Several studies have shown varying incidences of recovery, or progression to complete baldness, and the prognosis seems to differ pre- and

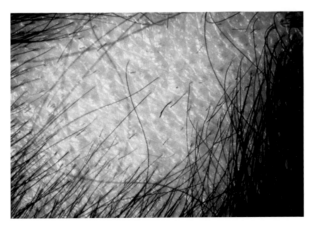

Figure 3.1
A typical patch of alopecia areata.

post-puberty. One study from Chicago reported that, of patients developing alopecia areata before puberty, 50% became totally bald and none recovered, while of those developing it after puberty only 25% became totally bald and 5.3% recovered. It also appears that alopecia areata occurring in atopic patients has a worse outcome.

Aetiology. The precise aetiology is uncertain, but a genetic predisposition appears to exist – family history increases the likelihood that a person will have the condition, and there are several reports of its occurrence in twins. Reports that alopecia areata is associated with autoimmune diseases, including thyroid disease, vitiligo and Addison's disease, have been interpreted as evidence for an autoimmune origin. Further evidence is the presence of a lymphocytic infiltrate in and around hair follicles of sufferers. Although antibodies that bind to extracts of human anagen hair follicles have been reported in the serum of patients with alopecia areata, similar antibodies are found in normal individuals, albeit at lower titres. However, alopecia areata differs from other recognized autoimmune diseases: it does not result in complete loss of function of the target organ, but rather in a temporary switching off of hair follicle activity, which can return to normal. This suggests that the target in alopecia areata may be a controlling growth factor or its receptor.

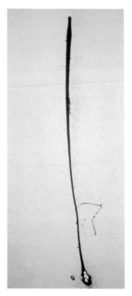

Figure 3.2 Exclamation-mark hair.

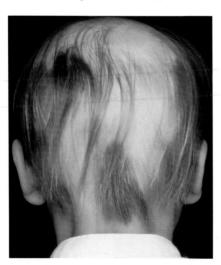

Figure 3.3 Moderately extensive alopecia areata.

Treatment. One of the main problems encountered when assessing the efficacy of any treatment for alopecia areata is the potential for natural recovery. To date, there is no completely reliable treatment and the majority of reports of therapeutic efficacy are anecdotal. Although the therapies described below can benefit some patients, many dermatologists prefer to adopt a 'wait-and-see' approach for this condition.

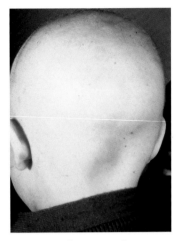

Figure 3.4 Alopecia totalis.

The earliest treatments were non-specific irritants; anecdotal accounts of improvement were related for phenol, benzylbenzoate, ultraviolet B light in erythematous doses, and dithranol. Supporting scientific evidence is, however, scant.

Steroids. Systemic corticosteroids result in regrowth of hair in many cases, but on discontinuing the treatment most patients relapse. Most investigators have felt that there was insufficient evidence of prolonged benefit to justify the potential systemic adverse reactions. Pulsed, intravenous prednisolone has been reported to prevent progression of recent-onset alopecia areata, though another study reported it to be ineffective in alopecia totalis. Some benefit was suggested in studies combining systemic steroids with topical or intralesional steroids, or topical minoxidil or cyclosporin, but the numbers of patients in these studies were small.

There have also been anecdotal reports of the effectiveness of topical corticosteroids, though regrowth of hair tends to occur in those cases in which it was most likely to have occurred spontaneously anyway; folliculitis may be a significant side-effect. Intralesional steroids administered either by needle or jet injection have been shown to be beneficial in some cases. Skin atrophy is an important side-effect which can occur not only at the site of injection but also in a linear fashion following the direction of lymph flow. Because of this, the intralesional steroids should be used principally for accelerating regrowth in well-circumscribed and cosmetically disfiguring areas of hair loss.

Sensitizers. Another approach has been the use of potent sensitizers to produce contact dermatitis, which may sometimes be associated with hair regrowth. Among the chemicals used for this purpose was dinitrochlorobenzene (DNCB). In one regimen, after sensitization was achieved using concentrations of up to 2%, once-weekly applications were applied at a concentration sufficient to achieve a mild inflammatory response (from concentrations as low as 0.0001%). Differing success rates were reported, ranging from 10 to 78%; the worst responses were seen in patients with alopecia totalis and those with a family history of alopecia areata and a personal or family history of atopy. However, following reports of potential carcinogenicity of DNCB, other sensitizing chemicals were studied, including squaric acid dibutyl ester (SADBE), *Primula obconica* and diphencyprone. The side-effects associated with induced dermatitis and the risk of sensitizing the medical staff administering the chemicals has led many dermatologists to abandon contact sensitization in the treatment of alopecia areata.

Psoralen and ultraviolet A. Some groups have reported that treatment with psoralen and ultraviolet A (PUVA), using oral 8-methoxypsoralen, is beneficial in up to 60% of cases. Again patients with alopecia totalis or atopy respond poorly. The exact mechanism of action is unknown, but may be due to the irritant effect of PUVA or the immunological changes that occur in the skin after PUVA treatment. Although some patients appear to respond well to PUVA, the overall poor response rate, high doses of UVA often required and high relapse rate has led many dermatologists to discontinue using it for alopecia areata.

Topical minoxidil was initially reported to be beneficial, though subsequent double-blind and dose-responsive studies were less encouraging.

Cyclosporin A. Oral cyclosporin A has been shown to produce hair regrowth in some cases, but it also induces general hypertrichosis, and renal and immunological side-effects. There have also been reports of its effectiveness when used in low doses with prednisolone, though other authors were unable to confirm this and have been reluctant to use it because of its toxicity.

Topical cyclosporin A has been tried in concentrations of 5–10%, and though it produced increased hair regrowth compared with placebo, this regrowth was patchy and sporadic.

FK506. Recent studies have shown that topical applications of the immunomodulatory drug FK506 (tacrolimus) can induce hair regrowth in a rat model of alopecia areata. This may prove to be an effective treatment for alopecia areata.

Trichotillomania

Patchy hair loss can occur as a consequence of trauma to the hair caused by rubbing or pulling. The physical clue is the presence of twisted and fragmented hairs, of normal colour and texture, broken at various distances from a clinically normal scalp. In children, it is usually the result of a hair-pulling habit, which can be confirmed on questioning the parents. In older patients with more extensive scalp involvement, the patient often denies touching his or her hair; it is frequently a manifestation of psychological disturbance, which is often difficult to correct, even with counselling and major and minor tranquillisers (Figure 3.5).

A similar pattern of trauma-induced patchy hair loss can be the consequence of traction during hairstyling (e.g. ponytails, plaiting, tight headwear and hot combing). Black African hair is particularly easily damaged by such procedures (Figure 3.6).

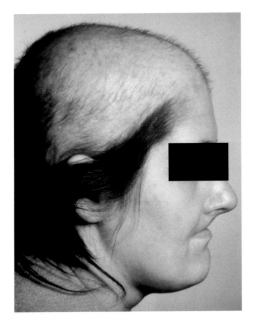

Figure 3.5
Trichotillomania.

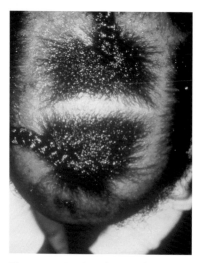

Figure 3.6 Traction alopecia due to plaiting.

Other causes

The presence of numerous small patches should raise the possibility of secondary syphilis and other clinical and serological evidence should be sought (Figure 3.7). Scaliness suggests a fungal infection and examination of the scalp using Wood's light or microscopy of scrapings and plucked hair helps to confirm this diagnosis.

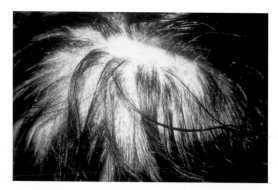

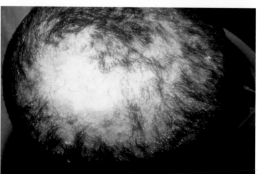

Figure 3.7 Hair loss due to secondary syphilis.

CHAPTER 4

Scarring hair loss

'Cicatricial', or scarring, is the general term applied to alopecia that accompanies or follows the permanent destruction of hair follicles, whether by a disease affecting the follicles themselves or by some external process. Follicles may be absent as the result of a developmental defect or may be irretrievably injured by trauma, as in the burns of radiodermatitis. They may be destroyed by a specific and identifiable infection – for example, favus, tuberculosis or syphilis – or by the encroachment of a tumour. In other cases, follicle destruction can be attributed to a named, though still cryptogenic, disease process such as lichen planus, lupus erythematosus (LE) or sarcoidosis.

When all the clinically and histologically acceptable causes have been eliminated, two named syndromes of cutaneous origin remain, pseudopelade and the less well-defined folliculitis decalvans. However, there are still some cases in which a diagnosis no more precise than 'cicatricial alopecia' can be made.

Assessment

On preliminary diagnosis of cicatricial alopecia, the scalp should be searched for other changes – folliculitis, follicular plugging or broken hairs – and hairs, even if grossly normal in appearance, should be extracted from the edge of the bald area for microscopy and culture. If no firm diagnosis is made, general skin examination should be performed for evidence of skin pathology elsewhere.

If the decision is made to take a biopsy, its site must be carefully selected and an early lesion is preferred. Several punch biopsies are preferable to a single elliptical biopsy because punch biopsies can be oriented along follicles and different stages of the disease process can be investigated.

The causes of cicatricial alopecia can be classified into an array of conditions. The more common causes are considered in the following section. For the many rarer entities, the reader is referred to more detailed texts.

Lupus erythematosus

Systemic LE does not usually cause scarring alopecia. More typically it causes diffuse shedding of hair, as in telogen effluvium, often during active, unstable phases of the disease.

However, discoid LE very often affects the scalp. The typical clinical appearance of discoid LE involving the scalp is an itchy, erythematous, scaly area, similar to discoid LE that occurs at other body sites, which extends irregularly and leaves scarring (Figure 4.1). However, in the absence of lesions elsewhere on the body, it may be difficult to differentiate discoid LE involving the scalp from pseudopelade or lichen planus. Histology at an early stage will show follicular plugging and basal liquefaction and a positive lupus band on immunofluorescence; in more advanced cases, histology may show only scarring.

Treatment with potent topical steroids may reduce erythema and inflammation and halt progression of the disease, but it may need to be supplemented with systemic corticosteroids and/or antimalarial agents. For cases that fail to respond to these measures, other therapies that have occasionally been used include dapsone, retinoids and oral gold. However, pharmacological measures cannot reverse scarring once it has occurred,

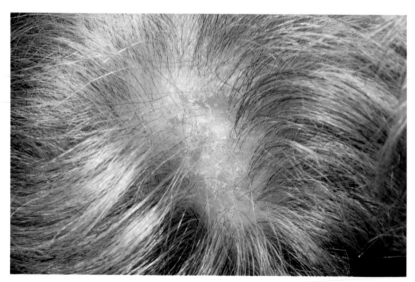

Figure 4.1 Scarring alopecia due to discoid lupus erythematosus.

though in cases where the disease has 'burnt out', surgical excision of scarred areas is an option.

Pseudopelade

In the 19th century, a pattern of slowly-progressing scarring alopecia with neither clinically evident folliculitis nor marked inflammation was described. This was termed 'pseudopelade'. There is no doubt that lichen planus can produce a very similar clinical picture and some authorities maintain, on the basis of associated skin lesions and histopathological findings, that 90% of pseudopelade cases are caused by lichen planus. At a later stage, LE can also cause similar changes. However, some patients with pseudopelade never show any clinical or histological evidence of lichen planus. Pseudopelade is therefore generally regarded as a clinical syndrome that may result from any one of a number of different pathological processes (known and unknown), though a clinically non-inflamed type has always been recognized.

Histologically, many lymphocytes can be found around the upper third of follicles in a clinically normal scalp at the edge of a plaque of pseudopelade. Later the follicles are destroyed and the epidermis becomes thin and atrophic, and the dermis densely sclerotic. Follicular 'ghosts' without inflammatory changes are seen.

Clinical features. Although both sexes may be affected, and the condition may occur in childhood, the patient is usually a woman over the age of 40 years. She may complain of slight scalp irritation at first, but more often a small bald patch or patches, discovered by chance by the patient or by her hairdresser, is the first evidence of disease. The initial patch is most often on the vertex, but may occur anywhere on the scalp (Figure 4.2). The course thereafter is extremely variable. In most cases, the condition develops only very slowly; indeed after 15 or 20 years the patient may still be able to arrange her hair to conceal bald patches effectively. In some cases, development occurs more rapidly, and exceptionally there may be almost total baldness after 2 or 3 years.

On examination, affected patches are smooth, soft and appear slightly depressed. At an early stage in the development of any individual patch there may be some erythema. The patches tend to be small and round or oval, but irregular bald patches may be formed by the confluence of many lesions.

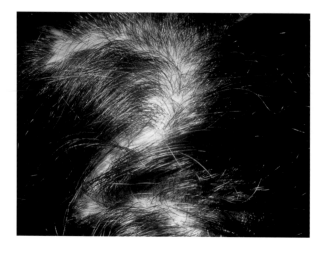

Figure 4.2
Pseudopelade.

TABLE 4.1

Diagnostic criteria for pseudopelade

Clinical

- Irregularly defined and confluent patches of alopecia
- Moderate atrophy (late stage)
- Mild perifollicular erythema (early stage)
- Female:male = 3:1
- Long course (more than 2 years)
- Slow progression, spontaneous termination possible

Direct immunofluorescence

- Negative, or at least only IgM

Histological

- Absence of marked inflammation
- Absence of widespread scarring
- Absence of significant follicular plugging
- Absence, or at least reduction, of sebaceous glands
- Presence of normal epidermis (only occasionally atrophy)
- Fibrotic streams into subcutis

The hair in uninvolved scalp is normal, but if the process is active, hairs at the edges of each patch are very easily extracted. Detailed clinical, histological and immunohistochemical examinations strongly support the idea that pseudopelade is a distinct entity with specific diagnostic criteria (Table 4.1).

Treatment. If scarring alopecia can be shown to be secondary to lichen planus or LE, then the treatment appropriate for these conditions may be prescribed. However, whether the baldness is of known or unknown origin, it is irreversible. If disfigurement is considerable and no active inflammatory changes are present, autografting from unaffected to scarred scalp, or surgical 'expansion' techniques in severe cases, may be considered.

Intradermal injection of corticosteroids does not seem to influence the extension of the disease process in cases of unknown origin.

Folliculitis decalvans

Under the general term 'folliculitis decalvans' we group together various syndromes in which clinically evident chronic folliculitis, often with overt pustulation, leads to progressive scarring (Figure 4.3). This is probably a heterogeneous group. Although the scalp is far and away the most commonly affected site, any or all hairy regions may be involved. There are multiple rounded or oval patches, each surrounded by crops of follicular pustules. There may be no other changes, but successive crops of pustules, each followed by destruction of the affected follicles, produce slow extension of the alopecia. The severity of the inflammatory changes fluctuates, but the course is prolonged.

Aetiology. The cause of folliculitis decalvans is still uncertain, but *Staphylococcus aureus* can almost always be grown from the pustules. Some abnormality of the host must be postulated. Some authors have emphasized the possible role of the seborrhoeic state and some use the term 'cicatrizing seborrhoeic eczema', but folliculitis decalvans is rare and the seborrhoeic state is common, so the association probably has no special significance.

It is possible that a local failure in the immune response or in leukocyte function may be the essential abnormality in most cases. Folliculitis decalvans of the scalp occurs in both sexes. It typically affects women aged 30–60 years, and men from adolescence onwards.

41

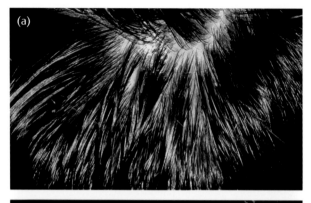

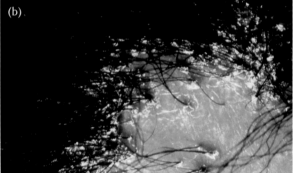

Figure 4.3
Folliculitis decalvans:
(a) in an early stage;
(b) at a later stage
of disease.

Tufted folliculitis may be a variant of this entity in which an upper follicular inflammatory infiltrate of polymorphs and some lymphocytes is clinically associated with close grouping or 'tufting' of hairs (Figure 4.4).

Treatment. All patients should be investigated for underlying defects of immune response and leukocyte function as a possible guide to effective treatment. Systemic antibiotics will often prevent further progression of disease, but only for as long as they are administered. Recent studies suggest that rifampicin with clindamycin is a useful combination. The effect of antibiotic treatment may be anti-inflammatory. Regular swabs should be taken for bacterial culture and sensitivity.

Lichen planus
Lichen planus is a disease or, more probably, a 'reaction pattern' of unknown origin that belongs to the autoimmune group of conditions.

It occurs worldwide, but there are marked regional variations in its incidence and clinical manifestations. These variations probably result from relative differences in the importance of various aetiological agents.

Pathology. The classical histology shows damage to the basal cells of the epidermis and an intense lymphocytic infiltrate in the upper dermis adjacent to the basement membrane. By immunofluorescence, fibrin and IgM may be detected in the upper dermis, and various components of complement are located in the basement membrane zone. If the process involves hair follicles, the infiltrate extends around them, particularly affecting the bulge area, and the lost hairs are replaced by keratin plugs. As the stem cell population (thought to be in the bulge area) appears to be affected, hair follicles may ultimately be totally destroyed.

Clinical features. Lichen planus occurs at any age, but in over 80% of cases the age at onset is between 30 and 70 years. Women are affected more often than men.

Early scalp lesions may show violaceous papules, erythema and scaling. As the disease progresses, follicular plugs become conspicuous and scarring replaces all other changes (Figure 4.5). The plugs are subsequently shed from the scarred areas, which remain white and smooth. If the patch is extending, horny plugs may still be present in follicles around its margins.

More often the scalp lesions are well established by the time the patient attends hospital and the irregular white patches are not clinically diagnostic, and indeed may not show any distinctive histological features. This clinical

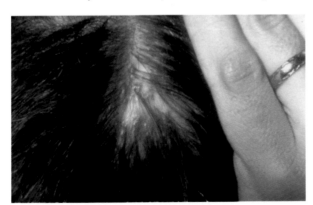

Figure 4.4
Tufted folliculitis.

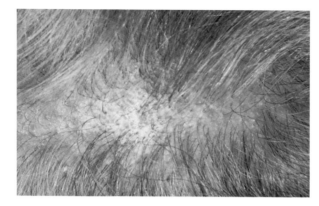

Figure 4.5
Lichen planus
of the scalp.

picture is often described as pseudopelade. Other rarer variants of lichen planus are the bullous (blistering), erosive and planopilaris forms. Diagnosis of lichen planus can be made only in the presence of unquestionable lesions elsewhere (e.g. mucous membranes or nails) and lichen planus histology.

Prognosis. In some patients, the course of lichen planus of the scalp is slow and after many years only a few inconspicuous patches are present. However, particularly if skin lesions are of the bullous or planopilaris type, they may rapidly result in extensive and permanent baldness. The rare childhood cicatricial lichen planus has a very poor prognosis.

Treatment. In some cases, in which there is active inflammation, scalp application of potent topical steroids, such as clobetasol propionate, twice daily may inhibit the process. In other cases, intralesional corticosteroids are helpful for treatment of active inflammation. However, for cases in which inflammation and scarring still progress despite topical and/or intralesional corticosteroids, systemic corticosteroids may be necessary.

Oral cyclosporin or azathioprine have been used in some cases, but their benefits are unreliable and both drugs have potentially hazardous side-effects.

Graham–Little syndrome (follicular lichen planus)

Whether this syndrome is a form of lichen planus, or not, is still unresolved, though immunofluorescent findings in typical cases strongly suggest lichen planus. Whatever its cause or causes, the syndrome is distinctive.

Most patients are women between 30 and 70 years of age. Essential features are progressive cicatricial alopecia of the scalp, loss of pubic and axillary hair without clinically evident scarring, and the development of horny follicular papules on the trunk, limbs and occasionally the eyebrows and sides of the face (follicular keratosis).

Biopsy of the scalp shows that the mouths of affected follicles are filled with horny plugs. The underlying follicle is progressively destroyed and eventually a thin epidermis covers scarred dermis. In the axillae and pubic region, the follicles are likewise destroyed, though clinically the skin does not appear to be atrophic.

No effective treatment is known, though surgical correction of scarring may be considered.

Frontal fibrosing alopecia

This condition, seen particularly in middle-aged or elderly women, is probably a variant of follicular scarring lichen planus. As the name implies it is a scarring alopecia that starts anteriorly and spreads posteriorly towards the vertex of the scalp (Figure 4.6). There is no effective pharmacological treatment once scarring has occurred, but application of a potent topical steroid to the margin may help slow its progression.

Circumscribed scleroderma (morphoea)

Circumscribed scleroderma rarely affects the scalp, but may occur there as single or multiple lesions. The early stages of morphoea appear as a lilac macule that slowly extends. Subsequently the centre becomes pearly or ivory white. Morphoea tends to regress spontaneously after 3–5 years, but may continue to extend for much longer. Hair is shed at an early stage to leave a cicatricial alopecia. Diagnosis must be confirmed histologically. Linear circumscribed morphoea in the frontal region may result in a depression in the contour of the scalp, which has led to the term 'coup de sabre' (Figure 4.7).

Cicatricial pemphigoid (benign mucosal pemphigoid/ocular pemphigus)

Cicatricial pemphigoid mainly affects the elderly, and women more than men. Bullae are formed at the dermo-epidermal junction. Linear deposits of IgG, C3 and C4 may be found in the basement membrane zone, but

45

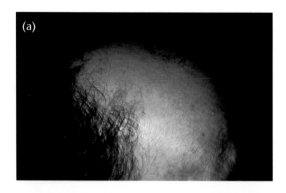

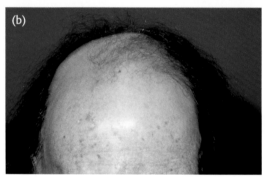

Figure 4.6
Frontal fibrosing alopecia: (a) viewed from the side; (b) viewed from the front.

circulating basement membrane zone antibodies (IgG or IgA) are not always demonstrable.

Disease affects the ocular and/or genital mucous membrane skin predominantly, but the skin is involved in 40–50% of cases. However, skin lesions may precede mucosal lesions by months or years, usual sites being the face and, in particular, the scalp. They recur repeatedly and leave dense scars.

Management is often dictated by the need to control the mucosal lesions. If recurrent bullae in a localized area of skin are troublesome, excision and grafting may be successful. Whether to prescribe oral corticosteroids or immunosuppressive drugs for skin lesions alone is controversial, but topical clobetasol propionate cream inhibits the process to some degree.

Erosive pustular dermatosis of the scalp

This clinical entity particularly affects women over 70 years of age. Its cause is unknown, but local trauma and sun-damage appear to be important

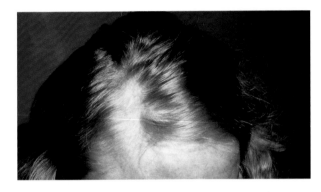

Figure 4.7
Morphoea (coup
de sabre).

causal factors. Initially a small area of scalp becomes red, crusted and
irritating. Crusting and superficial pustulation overlie a moist eroded surface
(Figure 4.8). As the condition extends, areas of activity co-exist with areas of
cicatricial alopecia. Squamous carcinoma may develop in the scars.

Differential diagnosis. Pyogenic and yeast infections are excluded by
bacteriological examination and by the lack of response to antibacterial
or antifungal agents. Biopsy may be necessary to exclude pustular psoriasis,
cicatricial pemphigoid, 'irritated' solar keratosis or squamous cell carcinoma.

Treatment. The stronger topical corticosteroids, such as 0.05% clobetasol
propionate twice daily, with occlusion if necessary, will suppress the

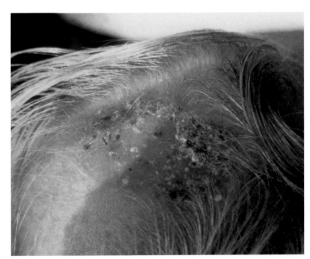

Figure 4.8
Erosive pustular
dermatosis of
the scalp.

inflammatory changes. It has been suggested that oral zinc sulphate may be curative in some cases.

Physical trauma

Physical injury to the scalp that damages hair follicles can result in scarring alopecia. Attachment of an electrode to the scalp for monitoring the fetal heartbeat during labour may occasionally cause some superficial damage to the scalp and this may be followed by a small scar. Aplasia cutis has sometimes been mistaken for such a lesion. Exceptionally, self-inflicted injuries may involve the scalp and leave scars.

Halo scalp ring

This type of alopecia, which may be temporary or permanent, is an area of scalp hair loss caused by prolonged pressure on the vertex by the uterine cervix during or prior to delivery, resulting in a haemorrhagic form of caput succedaneum.

Chronic radiodermatitis

X-ray epilation of the face for hirsutism was often employed during the first two decades of the 20th century. X-ray epilation for the treatment of scalp ringworm was introduced in Paris in 1904. The discovery of griseofulvin in 1958 gradually made X-ray epilation unnecessary, but it has been estimated that between 1904 and 1959 some 300 000 children worldwide were treated with X-rays for ringworm of the scalp. Correct dosage did not cause toxicity; however, technical errors were frequent, as apparatus was often inadequate and poorly calibrated. The treatment produced complete epilation in about 3 weeks and regrowth after 2 months. Follow up of those treated in childhood reveals a higher incidence of cancer in those who received treatment compared with a control group.

Radiodermatitis of the scalp may also occur as an unavoidable consequence of skin damage during treatment of both internal malignant disease and malignant disease of the skin.

Scarring due to developmental defects and hereditary disorders

Many syndromes characterized by keratosis pilaris, and associated with some degree of inflammatory change leading to destruction of affected follicles, have been described and elaborately named. All the conditions are assumed to be genetically determined, though many cases occur sporadically. Only detailed clinical and genetic studies can provide the facts essential for reliable differentiation of the syndromes that some authorities regard as forms or degrees of a single state while others regard as distinct entities. The reported cases can be conveniently classified into three groups, although additional rare well-defined entities have been reported.

Atrophoderma vermiculata (acne vermiculata, folliculitis ulerythematosa reticulata). Honeycomb atrophy of the cheeks occurs, as may scarring alopecia, though the latter is rare.

Keratosis pilaris atrophicans faciei (ulerythema oophryogenes). The process is more or less confined to the eyebrow region.

Keratosis pilaris decalvans (keratosis follicularis spinulosa decalvans, follicular ichthyosis). Keratosis pilaris of variable extent is associated with cicatricial alopecia.

Epidermolysis bullosa
The term 'epidermolysis bullosa' is applied to a group of distinct, genetically determined disorders characterized by the formation of bullae in the skin, and often also in the mucous membranes, either in response to trauma or spontaneously. Only one of these diseases is consistently accompanied by abnormalities of scalp or hair – recessive dystrophic epidermolysis bullosa. Alopecia may also occur in junctional epidermolysis bullosa.

CHAPTER 5

Ringworm

Tinea capitis is ringworm of the scalp in which the basic feature is invasion of hair shafts by a dermatophyte fungus. Most species of dermatophyte are capable of invading hair, but some species, such as *Microsporum audouinii* (the most common type of cat and dog origin), *Trichophyton schoenleinii* and *T. violaceum* have a particular predilection for the hair shaft. All dermatophytes causing scalp ringworm can invade glabrous skin and many attack nails as well. The species of dermatophyte fungus most likely to cause scalp fungal infection varies from country to country, and often from region to region. Moreover, in any given location the species may change with time, particularly as new organisms are introduced by immigration. It is of interest that in tinea capitis, anthropophilic species predominate.

In recent years, *M. canis* has become the dominant organism causing infections in Europe whereas *T. tonsurans* has spread through urban communities in the USA.

Pathogenesis

The spores of ringworm fungi causing tinea capitis can be found in the atmosphere close to the scalp of patients with the condition. It is highly likely that scalp hair acts as a trapping device, possibly enhanced by electrostatic forces. It is known that contamination of hair without any clinical findings may occur among classmates of children with tinea capitis. It is proven that, if actual hair infection is to develop, invasion of the stratum corneum of the scalp skin must first occur. Trauma assists inoculation, which is followed after approximately 3 weeks by overt hair-shaft infection. Spread to surrounding follicles proceeds for the period in which the infection persists, but it does not spread further. There is then a period of regression with or without an inflammatory phase.

Patterns of hair invasion

Two main patterns of tinea capitis are recognized – ectothrix and endothrix.

Ectothrix. The hyphae within the hair grow inwards towards the hair bulb, but at the same time other hyphae burst out through the hair surface, grow over the surface of the hair shaft and fragment into small spores (2–3 μm in diameter). This is the pattern seen in *Microsporum* species ('small spore ectothrix'). A similar pattern of invasion occurs with *T. mentagrophytes* and *T. verrucosum*, but the spores here are larger (3–5 μm and 5–10 μm diameter, respectively). The infected hair grows upwards and usually breaks off a few millimetres above the scalp surface.

Endothrix. The hyphae form spores within the cortex of the hair. Because of the greater degree of shaft damage, the hairs break off close to the scalp surface. This is the pattern of growth seen in *T. tonsurans*, *T. violaceum* and *T. soudanense*.

The favus types (e.g. *T. schoenleinii* and *T. quinckeanum*) also cause inflammatory changes in the epidermis and form scutula, which consist of spores and cellular debris in a dense network of mycelium.

Clinical features

The clinical appearance of ringworm of the scalp is quite variable. It depends on the type of hair invasion, level of host resistance and degree of inflammatory host response. The appearance, therefore, may vary from a few dull-grey broken-off hairs with a little scaling, detectable only on careful inspection, to a severe, painful inflammatory mass covering most of the scalp. In all types the main features are partial hair loss with some degree of inflammation. It is useful to recognize several basic clinical pictures.

Small-spored ectothrix infections. In *M. audouinii* and *M. ferrugineum* infections, the basic lesions are patches of partial alopecia often circular in shape, but showing broken-off hairs, which are dull-grey due to their coating of arthrospores. Inflammation is minor but fine scaling is characteristic, usually with a fairly distinct margin (Figure 5.1). There may be several or many patches arranged more or less randomly. In *M. canis* infection the picture is similar but there are more inflammatory changes. In infection caused by all these species, green fluorescence under Wood's lamp is usual but non-fluorescent cases have been reported. Children are affected much more often than adults, though the occasional case of tinea capitis in

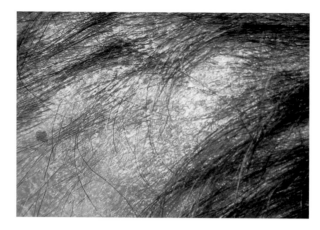

Figure 5.1
Fungal infection
of the scalp due
to small-spored
ectothrix infection.

older patients must not be forgotten. The attack rate for epidemic infections caused by anthropophilic species may be as high as 30% within a school class. In the past, infection rates of both *M. audouinii* and *M. canis* were much higher.

Kerion. The most severe pattern of reaction is known as a kerion (Figure 5.2). It is a painful inflammatory abscess-like mass in which such hairs as remain are loose. Follicles may discharge pus, there may be sinus formation and, on rare occasions, mycetoma-like grains may be found. Thick crusting with matting of adjacent hairs is common. The area affected may be limited, but multiple plaques can occur and occasionally a large confluent lesion may involve much of the scalp. Regional lymphadenopathy

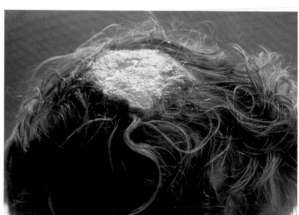

Figure 5.2
Kerion.

is common. Although this violent reaction is usually caused by one of the zoophilic species, typically *T. verrucosum* or *T. mentagrophytes*, occasionally a geophilic organism is isolated; anthropophilic infections that have been relatively inactive for weeks may suddenly become inflammatory and develop into kerions if a high degree of hypersensitivity develops. The possibility that secondary bacterial infection may play some part should not be ignored. In such cases a swab should be sent to the bacterial laboratory as well as sending plucked hairs for mycological assessment. Generally, however, pustule formation represents an inflammatory response to the fungus itself.

Endothrix infections. In *T. tonsurans* and *T. violaceum* infections, a relatively non-inflammatory type of patchy baldness occurs. Formation of black dots (swollen hair shafts) as the affected hair breaks at the surface of the scalp is a classical sign of this condition, but such findings may not be conspicuous. The patches, which are usually multiple, may show minimal scaling, sometimes mimicking discoid LE or seborrhoeic dermatitis. They are commonly angular rather than round in outline. A low-grade folliculitis is often seen, and sometimes a frank kerion may develop.

Favus. Infection with *T. schoenleinii* is seen sporadically in many countries, including South Africa, those of the Middle East, Pakistan, USA, UK and Australia. The classical picture of tinea capitis due to this organism is characterized by the presence of yellowish, cup-shaped crusts known as scutula. Each scutulum develops round a hair, which pierces it centrally. Adjacent crusts enlarge to become confluent, forming a mass of yellow crusting. Many patients may show less distinctive changes, in early cases perhaps amounting to no more than perifollicular redness and some matting of the hair. Extensive patchy hair loss with scarring alopecia and atrophy among patches of normal hair may be found in long-standing cases. In these patients, much of the hair loss is irreversible, and this has been hypothesized as being due to the destruction of the bulge area of the hair follicle. Some nail involvement is found in 2–3% of patients. Although initial infection probably occurs in childhood in nearly all cases, it shows little if any tendency to clear spontaneously at puberty, particularly in women. The existence of families with several affected generations has been reported.

Differential diagnosis

Tinea capitis must be distinguished from all conditions capable of causing patchy baldness with inflammatory changes of the scalp. Alopecia areata may show erythema, and though it is itself not a scaly condition, it may coexist with seborrhoeic dermatitis. Such cases can be confusing, though careful examination usually shows that the scaling and the hair loss are not co-extensive.

Exclamation-mark hair must be distinguished from the broken hairs of tinea capitis. Traumatic alopecia from hairdressing procedures and trichotillomania may also be confused. Seborrhoeic dermatitis is usually more diffuse than tinea capitis but in pityriasis ('tinea') amiantacea, the changes are often localized. In this condition, scaling is adherent to the hair, but breakage of the hair shaft does not normally occur. In psoriasis, hair loss is found only occasionally and again broken-off hairs are not usually present.

In impetigo, which may be secondary to pediculosis capitis, loosening of the hair is not normally present, but matting and crusting may cause confusion with inflammatory ringworm.

A carbuncle of the scalp is much more acutely painful, and typically causes systemic upset and fever, and shedding of loosened hair is much less evident than in kerion. Discoid LE, lichen planus and other causes of cicatricial alopecia may sometimes have to be considered.

Treatment

The mainstay of treatment in all these childhood conditions has, for many years, been griseofulvin. Topical therapy has little place in the management of this condition except as an adjunct to oral therapy, though it is sensible to remove matted crusts and to carry out routine frequent shampooing. Although massive, single-dose griseofulvin therapy and intermittent dose schedules (e.g. 25 mg/kg, twice a week) have had some success, in general it is advisable to use the conventional treatment with griseofulvin 10 mg/kg per day, given once daily or divided into two doses. In small-spore ectothrix infections, griseofulvin, 10 mg/kg per day for 4–6 weeks, is usually adequate. Where possible, infected hair should be clipped away to reduce the infectivity of the patient.

At present, the newer azole and allylamine antifungals, such as terbinafine and itraconazole, though effective against many fungi capable of infecting the scalp, are not licensed for use in children.

Control

It is of considerable importance with scalp ringworm to discover the species involved. Some information may be obtained from the clinical picture or the presence or absence of fluorescence, but culture is required for a diagnosis to be accurately established. Where animal species are concerned, the source should be proved mycologically: it is not always the expected one. The course of action to be taken depends upon the situation and the value placed upon the animal. A small, much-loved domestic pet can often be treated successfully and economically with griseofulvin. Cattle ringworm in calves will normally settle spontaneously. A group of highly infected laboratory mice should probably be destroyed.

With anthropophilic infections, careful investigation of the outbreak or epidemic is recommended and exclusion of children from school is probably necessary. Apart from the risk of spreading infection, there is often a sound sociological basis for keeping an infected child at home. It demonstrates social awareness and responsibility by the family and avoids a situation in which the family may be accused of spreading infection. With zoophilic infections such as *M. canis*, children can normally be allowed to remain at school as human-to-human infectivity is low.

CHAPTER 6

Hirsuties in women

Hirsuties affecting women may be defined as growth of terminal hair on the body of a woman in the same pattern as that which develops in the normal postpubertal male. However, the perception of hirsuties is, by definition, subjective and women present with wide variation in the degree of severity. Acceptance of hirsuties by the patient is influenced by cultural and social factors (Figure 6.1).

Hirsuties is often seen in endocrinological disorders associated with hyperandrogenism (Table 6.1). These disorders may include abnormalities of the ovaries or adrenal glands. The majority of women have polycystic ovary

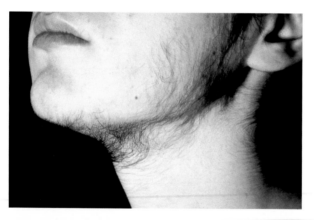

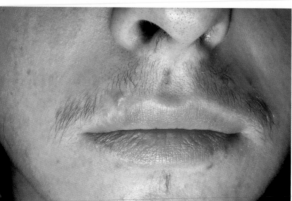

Figure 6.1
Hirsuties in premenopausal women.

TABLE 6.1

Causes of hirsuties

- Ovarian causes
  - polycystic ovary syndrome
  - ovarian tumours
- Adrenal causes
  - congenital adrenal hyperplasia
  - adrenal tumours
- Cushing's disease
- Prolactinoma
- Gonadal dysgenesis
- Androgen therapy
- Idiopathic hirsuties
- ??Obesity

syndrome and only a small proportion have a serious endocrinological disorder. A small proportion of hirsute women have no detectable hormone abnormality and are usually classified as idiopathic. However, with improving endocrine assays, the subgroup of idiopathic patients is becoming smaller as increasing numbers of hirsute women can be shown to have subtle forms of ovarian or adrenal hypersecretion, or altered androgen-binding proteins or cutaneous metabolism of androgens. Although many hirsute women are obese, the role of adipose tissue is poorly defined. It is clinically recognized that in many hirsute women, weight loss can improve any menstrual irregularity and reduce hirsutism.

Diagnostic approach

History should include duration of hirsuties, other features of cutaneous androgen effects, such as acne vulgaris or androgenetic alopecia, and evidence of polycystic ovary syndrome such as irregular menses or infertility. A family history of childhood dehydration or precocious puberty in a brother might suggest congenital adrenal hyperplasia, and galactorrhoea might indicate excessive prolactin production. A drug history should be

57

taken to exclude an ingested source of androgens such as glucocortico-steroids or anabolic steroids. The progestogenic component of many contraceptive preparations are relatively androgenic and are often cited as a cause of hirsuties, though in practice this effect is not usually relevant.

Physical examination should include the pattern and severity of the hair growth, associated androgenetic alopecia, acne vulgaris, obesity, acanthosis nigricans, deepening of the voice, increased muscle bulk, hypertension, galactorrhoea, striae distensae and cliteromegaly. Cliteromegaly is the most important sign pointing towards systemic virilization; if it is associated with a short history of onset of hirsutism (less than 1 year), it is highly suggestive of a tumorous cause.

Investigations. The following recommendations for investigation are those used by many specialists dealing with hirsuties.
- Long-standing mild hirsuties with regular menstrual cycle and no features of systemic virilism. No further investigation required.
- Moderate hirsuties with or without menstrual irregularities. The majority of these patients have polycystic ovary disease, which may be confirmed on ultrasound examination; a plasma testosterone assay may be helpful. These patients only require further investigations if they fail to improve with adequate anti-androgen therapy.
- Severe hirsuties and virilization with a short history, or very severe hirsuties with a long history should be thoroughly investigated for an androgen-secreting tumour.

Treatment
Cosmetic approaches include bleaching, shaving (there is no evidence that shaving stimulates hair growth despite popular belief), plucking (e.g. waxing or sugaring) and depilatory creams (though these can result in redness and soreness). Electrolysis is the only permanent method of hair removal, but it can be painful. At present, lasers are unable to achieve permanent hair loss reliably.

Systemic anti-androgen drugs can be helpful. Cyproterone acetate and spironolactone are the two most often prescribed. Several dose regimens of cyproterone acetate have been used.

Low-dose therapy is frequently given as the contraceptive pill Dianette® (Diane 35 ED, Schering Healthcare; currently unavailable in the USA), which contains 35 µg ethinyloestradiol and 2 mg cyproterone acetate, taken for 21 days in 28. Some clinicians use hormone-replacement therapy as a treatment for hirsuties in menopausal and postmenopausal women to reduce free androgen, though there are no published studies to support its use.

High-dose therapy consists of Dianette® for 21 days, with cyproterone acetate, 50–100 mg, for the first 10 days only (the reverse sequential regimen of Hammerstein). However, some dose-ranging studies have suggested that there is no major dose effect. For example, a large multicentre study performed in Canada reported that, after 12 months' treatment, the mean reduction in hirsuties score with Diane® (Schering Healthcare), which contains 2 mg cyproterone acetate and 50 µg ethinyloestradiol, was 25% whereas with Diane plus 100 mg cyproterone acetate, the reduction was only marginally better at 31%.

Spironolactone has been used at doses ranging from 50 to 200 mg taken either daily or cyclically (daily for 3 weeks in every 4). A daily dose of 200 mg has been reported to produce a reduction in subjective hair growth of approximately 40% after 6 months' therapy. At doses below that there are conflicting reports of efficacy. Open and blind studies comparing spironolactone and cyproterone acetate have suggested that there are few differences between the two therapies. Spironolactone may feminize a male fetus, and consequently pregnancy should be avoided while taking it.

Other agents. Cimetidine was initially reported as being beneficial but subsequent studies have not confirmed this. Finasteride has been reported to be useful, but has not received a licence for use in women at the time of press because of its feminizing effects on the male fetus. Although flutamide and ketoconazole have also reduced hirsutism, they should be avoided because of the risk of hepatic toxicity.

CHAPTER 7

Scaly scalp

Pityriasis capitis (pityriasis simplex, furfuracea, dandruff)

This near-physiological scaling of the scalp is most common at about the age of 20 years, when it is estimated that up to half the Caucasian population develop it. The aetiology is uncertain, but the peak incidence at this age suggests an androgenic influence. The role of *Pityrosporum ovale (Malassezia furfur)* has been debated for many years: while evidence for its role is that application of yeast inhibitors produces a reduction in pityriasis, other authors consider that the increased numbers of *P. ovale* in pityriasis capitis is a secondary effect of the increased scaling.

Treatment with selenium sulphide (which has been shown to reduce epidermal turnover time), or zinc pyrithione or zinc omadine (which are said to reduce yeast populations), is usually effective in most, but not all, patients. Those authors who have proposed a role for yeasts have suggested treatment with imidazole compounds (e.g. shampoo containing ketoconazole). In patients with more severe pityriasis, particularly if associated with seborrhoea, a tar preparation rubbed into involved areas on the scalp and washed out after a few hours with a tar shampoo may be effective.

Seborrhoeic dermatitis

Pityriasis capitis is regarded by many as the mildest form of seborrhoeic dermatitis, which is characterized by erythematous flaky areas that are often associated with greasy yellowish scales (Figure 7.1). The hairline and postauricular areas are most often involved, and the eyebrows, nasolabial folds and sternum can also be affected.

Treatment. For mild seborrhoeic dermatitis azole shampoos (e.g. ketoconazole) or 2% fluconazole shampoo are often effective and the scalp should be shampooed twice or more each week until the condition is under control. If the seborrhoeic dermatitis is severe, a topical preparation

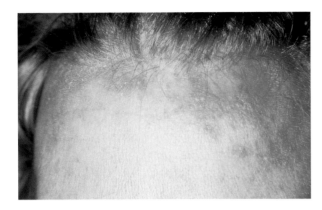

Figure 7.1
Seborrhoeic
dermatitis.

containing tar and sulphur or Oil of Cade ointment should be rubbed gently
into the scalp at least two hours before shampooing. For the erythema of
severe seborrhoeic dermatitis a daily application of a moderately potent
topical steroid can be helpful. If secondary infection is present a topical
antibiotic–corticosteroid combination should be prescribed and if secondary
infection is severe extensive systemic antibiotics may be required. Some
clinicians have suggested that topical lithium succinate is also a safe and
effective treatment in seborrhoeic dermatitis. The condition has a tendency
to recur so some patients prefer to use an azole shampoo on a regular basis
to prevent relapse.

Psoriasis

Scalp involvement in psoriasis is common and indeed the scalp may be the
initial site of involvement. The presence of typical psoriasis elsewhere on the
body or nails aids the diagnosis and sometimes the scalp remains continually
involved for many years while lesions elsewhere on the body come and go.
The clinical spectrum of scalp psoriasis ranges from pink plaques covered in
a silvery scale resembling those seen in other parts of the body (Figure 7.2),
to patchy scaling, or at the other end of the clinical spectrum, layers of
asbestos-like scale (pityriasis amiantacea) (Figure 7.3). Hair loss may occur
but is usually reversible. Rarely, very severe disease can result in scarring
alopecia.

Treatment. In mild cases, treatment with a tar-based or keratolytic shampoo
is sufficient. Topical calcipotriol may also prove effective in milder cases.

61

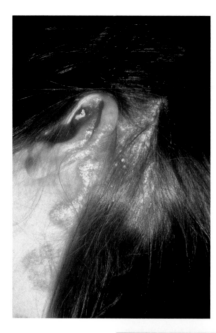

Figure 7.2 Scalp psoriasis.

Figure 7.3 Pityriasis amiantacea.

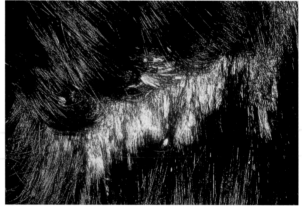

More severe cases often respond well to a topical keratolytic agent, such as Cocois or arachis oil, left on for a few hours then washed off using a tar-based shampoo (patients often find it most effective to apply the treatment at night, cover with a plastic shower cap or scarf while asleep, and then wash it off in the morning). Treatment should be performed every evening until the scalp is clear – this usually takes 7–10 days. Once the scalp is clear maintenance can be achieved by repeating this treatment either once weekly or once fortnightly, or alternatively by washing with Capasal shampoo (containing 1% distilled coal tar, 0.5% salicylic acid and 1% coconut oil) once weekly.

If this treatment regimen is ineffective Oil of Cade ointment can be used instead – rubbed in at night and washed off in the morning. An alternative is dithranol pommade massaged into the scalp taking care to avoid contact with the eyes and washed off after 2–4 hours. The disadvantages of dithranol pommade are that it can burn the scalp if left on for longer than this and it can also stain blonde hair.

For associated erythema, a topical steroid preparation, such as Betnovate® lotion (Glaxo Wellcome) or Synalar® gel (Bioglan), applied once or twice daily, can be helpful. However, topical steroids alone are ineffective against thick scale which requires keratolytic agents too.

CHAPTER 8
'Funny-looking' hair in children

Hair problems in children present relatively often. While disorders such as alopecia areata, tinea capitis and trichotillomania account for most of these, there are a significant number of congenital and hereditary causes of hair problems that can occur. Usually these hair disorders are isolated abnormalities and the child is otherwise well, although this is not always the case. A number of hair disorders occur as part of a multisystem syndrome and recognition of the hair disorder may enable diagnosis of that syndrome.

Childhood hair disorders can be broadly categorized into two groups:
- those where there are fewer hairs on the scalp
- those that involve production of an abnormal hair fibre.

Decreased hair production will present with sparse or absent hair, while abnormal hair fibre production may produce either unruly hair, spangled hair, hair that has an unusual texture, or weak hairs that readily break off to produce areas of hair loss covered with a stubble of short broken hairs.

Not all congenital or hereditary hair disorders are present at birth, and those that are often go unnoticed. This is because many normal children are born without much hair and remain without much hair during the first year of life, making sparse hair during this period unremarkable.

There appear to be some differences between the early, synchronized hair growth of infancy and the non-synchronized hair growth of children and adults (see Chapter 1). Some so-called congenital disorders do not present until childhood as they spare the synchronized hairs. In addition, latent gene expression also delays presentation of a number of hereditary disorders characterized by programmed destruction of the follicles, such as Marie Unna syndrome.

Hypotrichosis
Hereditary hypotrichosis and atrichia congenita. In hereditary hypotrichosis there is a profound reduction in the number of hair follicles on the scalp usually, but not always, from birth. Atrichia congenita refers to a condition where there is total and permanent absence of scalp hair. It may begin at birth, or be delayed for up to 5 years. It needs to be distinguished from

alopecia areata totalis, for which a biopsy from the scalp may be required. On biopsy there may be evidence of follicular agenesis or programmed destruction of the hair follicles with scarring.

Both autosomal dominant and autosomal recessive pedigrees have been described, and atrichia congenita may occur as an isolated phenomenon or associated with:

- facial papular cysts
- immunodeficiency
- epilepsy and mental retardation
- deafness
- ocular abnormalities
- ichthyosis
- skeletal abnormalities
- inborn errors of metabolism
- premature ageing syndromes, such as progeria.

Marie Unna syndrome. Dr Marie Unna first described this autosomal dominant disorder in 27 affected members of a family over seven generations. The hair may be normal at birth or sparse. During the third year it becomes coarse and twisted, resembling an ill-fitting wig. With the approach of puberty, the hair is progressively lost from the scalp (initially over the vertex) due to destruction of the follicles with scarring (Figure 8.1).

Ectodermal dysplasia defines a group of inherited developmental syndromes with disorders in more than one ectoderm-derived tissue. The defect presumably manifests during early embryological development, some time after the third week post-conception, when ectoderm can first be distinguished from mesoderm and endoderm, but before the end of the third month, when ectodermal cells have become committed to differentiate into specific derivative structures.

Ectodermal cells during this period (between 3 weeks and 3 months) have the potential to develop into either neuroectoderm or surface ectoderm (Figure 8.2).

Any developmental abnormality that damages ectodermal cells in this window period prior to committed differentiation may result in abnormalities in the infant in a large number of organs. In general, those

(a)

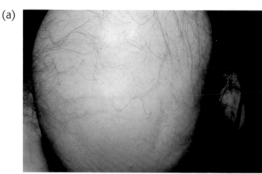

Figure 8.1

Marie Unna syndrome:
(a) typical appearance of
scalp vertex in a young
adult; (b) view of
posterior scalp.

(b)

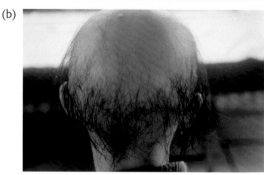

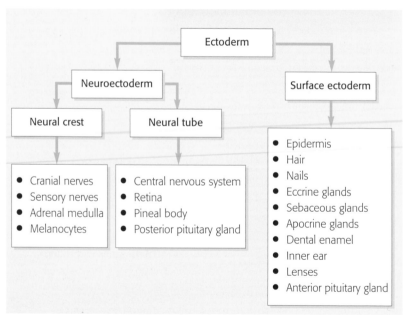

Figure 8.2 Tissues derived from ectoderm.

fetuses that survive often manifest abnormalities of hair, nails, epidermis, teeth and eccrine glands. These abnormalities (Table 8.1) form the basis of classification for ectodermal dysplasias (Table 8.2).

TABLE 8.1

Manifestations of abnormal development of surface ectoderm-derived tissues

Hair

- Alopecia
- Follicular atrophoderma
- Hair shaft structural abnormalities
- Hypotrichosis
- Keratosis pilaris

Nails

- Anonychia
- Non-specific dysplasia
- Thickening

Epidermis

- Abnormal dermatoglyphics
- Blisters
- Cleft lip and palate
- Excessive bruising and scarring
- Ichthyosis
- Palmar keratoses
- Palmar-plantar keratoderma
- Xerosis or poikiloderma

Apocrine glands

- Absent nipple or areola
- Mammary hypoplasia
- Supernumerary nipples

Eccrine glands

- Defective sweating
- Impaired thermoregulation

Teeth

- Abnormal dentition
- Enamel defects with premature loss
- Failure of dental eruption
- Gingival hyperplasia
- Peg-shaped incisors

Ears

- Abnormal or malformed auricles
- Folded or floppy ears
- Low-set ears
- Prominent ears
- Sensorineural deafness

Eyes

- Cataracts
- Corneal dyskeratosis or scarring
- Corneal opacities
- Decreased lacrimation
- Entropion
- Glaucoma
- Iris atrophy
- Keratoconus
- Nystagmus
- Photophobia

TABLE 8.2

An abbreviated list of the ectodermal dysplasias associated with abnormalities of the hair (modified from Olsen, 1994)

Ectodermal dysplasia	Inheritance*	Hair
Anhidrotic (Christ, Siemens, Touraine)	XLR	Sparse, pale, fine, short, increases at puberty
Hypohidrotic	AR	Sparse, pale, fine, short
Rapp–Hodgkin syndrome	AD	Sparse, pale, like steel wool
Ectrodactyly, cleft lip and palate (EEC)	AD	Sparse, light, wiry
Ankyloblepharon, cleft lip and palate	AD	Fine, wiry, sparse or absent
Keratosis, ichthyosis, deafness (KID) syndrome	?AD	Diffuse, fine, sparse or absent; improves with time
Pachyonychia congenita	AD	Generalized hypotrichosis in >10% and kinky hair
Focal dermal hypoplasia (Goltz syndrome)	XL	Sparse, brittle hair and focal areas of aplasia cutis
ANOTHER syndrome	AR	Hypotrichosis and brittle hair
Hidrotic (Clouston)	AD	Sparse, fine, pale or absent
Trichorhinopharyngeal syndromes I and II	AD or AR	Sparse, pale, brittle hair and temporal alopecia
Freid's tooth and nail syndrome	AR	Marked hypotrichosis, twisting
Schopf–Schultz–Passarge syndrome	AR	Marked hypotrichosis

*AR, autosomal recessive; AD, autosomal dominant; XLR, X-linked recessive; XLD, X-linked dominant

Conical teeth	Nail dystrophy	Decreased sweating	Associated features
+	+	+	Distinctive facies, absent nipples, recurrent upper respiratory tract infections
+	+	+	The sweating defect is less severe than in the XLR form
+	+	+	Distinctive facies, deafness ± syndactyly
+	+	+	Lobster-claw hand, cleft lip and palate
+	+	+	Syndactyly, abnormal ears, eyes and nipples
+	+	+	Distinctive facies, blindness, ichthyosis, deafness
+	+	+	Grossly thickened nails, palmar-plantar keratoderma with bullae, keratosis pilaris, leukoplakia, warts
+	+	+	Limb asymmetry, syndactyly, ectrodactyly, focal dermal hypoplasia, eye abnormalities
+	+	+	Clinodactyly, syndactyly, hypothyroidism, ephelides, cardiovascular, respiratory and gastro-intestinal abnormalities
+	+	±	Keratoderma, patchy hyperpigmentation, cataracts, clubbing
+	+	−	Abnormal facies, brachiopharyngeal dystosis, high arched palate, hyperextensible joints
+	+	−	Abnormal facies, cleft lip, branchial neck cyst
+	+	−	Follicular hyperkeratosis, palmar–plantar keratoderma, eyelid apocrine hidrocystomas

TABLE 8.2 (continued)

An abbreviated list of the ectodermal dysplasias associated with abnormalities of the hair (modified from Olsen, 1994)

Ectodermal dysplasia	Inheritance*	Hair
Schinzel–Giedion syndrome	AR	Generalized hypertrichosis
Coffin–Siris syndrome	AD	Hypotrichosis scalp, limbs, back and face
Cranioectodermal syndrome	AR	Thin, short and very fine
Incontinentia pigmenti	XLD	Hypotrichosis and linear alopecia
Benign atrophic epidermolysis bullosa	AR?	Thin and lustreless hair, scarring alopecia
Congenital insensitivity to pain	AR	Hypotrichosis
Alopecia-onychodysplasia-hypohidrosis syndrome	?	Universal alopecia
Alopecia-onychodysplasia-hypohidrosis	?	Severe generalized hypotrichosis
Orofacial digital syndrome	XLD	Fine, dry, sparse
Hallermann–Streiff syndrome	AD or AR	Generalized hypotrichosis, focal alopecia, absent brows
Sabina's brittle hair and mental deficiency	AR	Sparse, dry, coarse, weathered hair
Trichofacial hypohidrotic syndrome	XLR	Sparse, brittle hair

*AR, autosomal recessive; AD, autosomal dominant; XLR, X-linked recessive; XLD, X-linked dominant

Conical teeth	Nail dystrophy	Decreased sweating	Associated features
+	+	−	Telangiectasia, simian creases, abnormal facies, skeletal, renal and cardiac abnormalities, mental and growth retardation
+	+	−	Abnormal facies, absent fifth terminal metacarpal, skeletal and cardiac abnormalities, eczema, peptic ulcer
+	+	−	Abnormal facies, hypotonia, rhizomelia, syndactyly, clinodactyly, osteoporosis, cardiac abnormalities
+	+	−	Infantile blisters, later linear verrucous lesions and whorled pigmentation, CNS and retinal abnormalities, cleft lip and palate
+	+	−	Traumatic blisters from birth, no secondary sexual hair, palmar-plantar keratoderma, eye abnormalities
+	−	+	Universal sensory loss, Charcot's joints, pseudoainhum
−	+	+	Eczema, photophobia, epilepsy, nystagmus, hypospadias, mental retardation
−	+	+	Deafness, palmar-plantar keratoderma, photophobia, estropia
+	−	−	Mental retardation, facial, oral and skeletal abnormalities, cleft lip and palate, syndactyly, polydactyly, brachydactyly
+	−	−	Mental retardation, cataracts, focal cutaneous atrophy, cardiac abnormalities
−	+	−	Abnormal facies, mental retardation, retinal abnormalities, scalp hyperkeratosis
−	−	+	Abnormal facies, upper respiratory problems

Other abnormalities that may occur include deafness, mental retardation, breast hypoplasia, cleft lip and palate, syndactyly, skeletal abnormalities and distinctive facies. Bony abnormalities, though reflecting an abnormality of mesenchyme-derived tissues, do not exclude diagnosis of ectodermal dysplasia.

In order to fulfil the criteria for an ectodermal dysplasia, there must be a congenital, non-progressive abnormality in at least two ectoderm-derived tissues.

Alopecia areata totalis may begin at any age, though onset in infancy is exceptional. Unless there is a classical evolution of circular patches with exclamation-mark hairs to total alopecia, a biopsy should be performed to distinguish this condition from congenital and hereditary causes of hair loss.

Abnormal hair fibre production
Abnormal hair fibre production may produce unruly hair, spangled hair, fragile hair or hair that feels different. It is produced by a small number of disorders, which are discussed in detail at the end of this chapter.

Unruly hair. Hair may be unruly because it is twisted, curled or irregularly shaped. Normal European hair is circular or ellipsoid and regular in size and shape. Akin to stacking a wood pile, the regular ellipsoid hairs sit easily together. Irregularly shaped hair or hair that is twisted or curled is more difficult to 'stack together'.

Conditions that give rise to unruly hair include:
- uncombable hair (cheveux incoiffables)
- pili torti
- woolly hair.

Spangled hair. Hair twists reflect the light at various angles and produce a spangled appearance. Hair with alternating light and dark bands also has a spangled appearance.

Conditions in which a spangled appearance is seen include:
- pili torti
- twisting hair dystrophy
- pili annulati
- monilethrix (occasionally).

Areas of hair loss covered with a stubble of broken-off hairs. On average, hairs grow at the rate of 1 cm per month. Thus the tip of a hair that is 36 cm long has been exposed to the environment for almost 3 years. During that period it is likely to have been washed and dried over 500 times, combed or brushed countless times and perhaps bleached, dyed or permed as well. Consequently, the tip of the hair will show signs of deterioration. While a normal hair will show the scars of these procedures, collectively known as 'weathering', it will survive this onslaught. On the other hand, a hair that has a structural weakness that renders it fragile will not and is likely to split and snap off. The amount of weathering hair can withstand will determine how long a hair grows before it breaks. This in turn will be determined by the nature and severity of the intrinsic structural weakness.

Many of the conditions associated with weak hair fibres are caused by single gene defects. A number of these genodermatoses can be diagnosed by examination of the fibres by light microscopy as they produce specific deformities.

Conditions that result in areas of hair loss covered with a stubble of broken-off hairs include:
- monilethrix
- pili torti
- twisting hair dystrophy
- Netherton's syndrome
- trichothiodystrophy
- regrowing alopecia areata
- trichotillomania
- tinea capitis.

Less commonly it can arise from:
- hypothyroidism
- anaemia
- malnutrition
- connective tissue disorders.

Hair with an unusual texture. Hair consists of a cortex and central medulla surrounded by a proteinaceous cuticle. The cuticle is, in turn, surrounded by a hydrophobic lipid envelope, which gives hair its lustre and silky texture. The first changes induced by hair weathering are loss of the lipid exocuticle and the cuticle itself. This gives rise to a limp, lustreless appearance and a coarse texture.

In loose anagen syndrome, hair has an unusual tacky feel to it that is quite distinctive. The cause is unknown, though preliminary investigations suggest that the composition of the lipid envelope is abnormal.

Specific hair shaft disorders

Uncombable hair (cheveux incoiffables). This is an autosomal dominantly inherited genodermatosis, characterized by triangular hairs. The hair is first noticed to be abnormal at about the age of 3 years. While normal in quantity and length, it is unruly and resists all attempts to control it with a brush or comb (Figure 8.3). The pathognomonic feature seen on light and electron microscopy is that more than 50% of the hairs have a triangular or kidney-shaped cross-section with a longitudinal groove running along almost the entire length of the hair.

Pili torti. With this disorder, the hairs are flattened and twisted through 180° at irregular intervals along the shaft. The hairs are also fragile and snap off when handled roughly. Not all hairs are affected and the proportion of affected hairs varies from person to person, even within families (Figure 8.4).

The twisting gives the hair a spangled appearance, and the fragility may lead to circumscribed areas of baldness at sites of friction and trauma. In severe cases there may be only short coarse stubble over the entire scalp

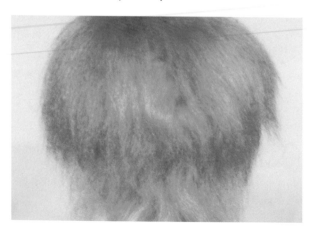

Figure 8.3
Uncombable hair.

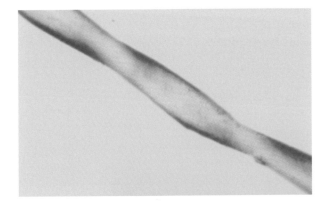

Figure 8.4
Appearance of pili torti hair under the light microscope.

Figure 8.5
Clinical appearance of the scalp of a patient with pili torti.

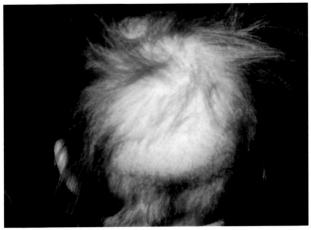

(Figure 8.5). In areas not subjected to trauma, where the hair is allowed to grow long, the twisting renders it unruly.

The natural history of pili torti is variable. In the classic form, the hair is normal at birth and is gradually replaced by spangled blonde abnormal hair between the third month and the third year. The hair remains abnormal until puberty when it darkens in colour, becomes less fragile and grows to an acceptable length.

Pili torti is also a feature of:

- Menke's syndrome (X-linked recessive with low serum copper levels and mental retardation)
- Björnstad's syndrome (autosomal dominant with sensorineural deafness)

75

TABLE 8.3

Syndromes associated with pili torti

Syndrome	Features
Menke's kinky hair	• Pale skin and progressive psychomotor retardation syndrome due to an X-linked inborn error of copper transportation
Björnstad's syndrome	• Autosomal dominant condition with sensorineural deafness
Bazex syndrome	• Basal cell carcinoma and follicular atrophoderma
Conradi–Hunermann syndrome	• Chondrodysplasia punctata, limb asymmetry, characteristic facies, spontaneously resolving congenital ichthyosiform erythroderma, hypotrichosis, cicatricial alopecia, follicular atrophoderma, limb asymmetry, abnormal nails and cataracts
Crandall's syndrome	• Sex-linked with deafness and hypogonadism
Citrullinaemia	• Hereditary arginosuccinic acid synthetase deficiency
Trichothiodystrophy	• Ichthyosis, photosensitivity, brittle sulphur-deficient hair, mental and growth retardation, neutropenia and decreased fertility
Salti–Salem syndrome	• Hypogonadotrophic hypogonadism
Some ectodermal dysplasias	• Characteristic facies, nail, sweating and dental defects
	• Salamon syndrome
	• Arthrogryphosis and ectodermal dysplasia
	• Ectodermal dysplasia with syndactyly
	• Tricho-odonto-onycho-dysplasia with syndactyly
	• Pili torti and enamel hypoplasia
	• Pili torti and onychodysplasia
	• Rapp–Hodgkin's syndrome
	• Ankyloblepharon-ectodermal dysplasia-cleft lip and palate (AEC) syndrome

- Bazex syndrome (multiple basal cell carcinomas and follicular atrophoderma)
- Crandall's syndrome (X-linked recessive with deafness and hypogonadism)
- a number of ectodermal dysplasias (Table 8.3).

Twisting hair dystrophy. There are a number of disorders where the hair is irregularly twisted. Half and three-quarter twists may be seen rather than the full 180° twists seen in true pili torti. These twists are non-specific and occur in a number of heterogeneous disorders and ectodermal dysplasias. Acquired twisting is also almost invariably seen at the edge of a scarring alopecia. In such cases the twisting is due to follicular distortion by the scarring process.

Woolly hair is tightly coiled hair over all or part of the scalp resembling Negroid hair, but occurring in a person not of Negroid origin. Localized, naevoid woolly hair is present at birth and appears not to be genetically determined (Figure 8.6). In contrast, generalized woolly hair is inherited either as an autosomal dominant trait or an autosomal recessive trait.

The hairs are fine and of irregular calibre with occasional loose twists. Hair may be fragile, but this is not usually very pronounced.

An acquired form of woolly hair also exists, but this appears to be a distinct condition that is usually a precursor of androgenetic alopecia.

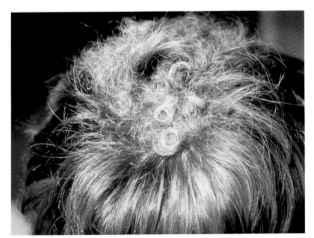

Figure 8.6
Woolly hair naevus.

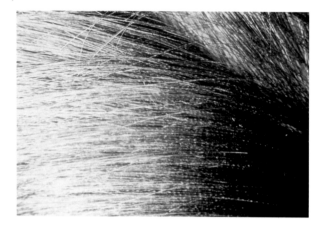

Figure 8.7
Spangled appearance of scalp due to pili annulati.

Pili annulati. Patients rarely present with pili annulati and it is more an incidental finding. Patches of hair on the scalp have a spangled appearance due to the alternating light and dark bands that occur in this autosomal dominant condition (Figure 8.7).

The alternating light and dark bands are also seen on light microscopy. The light bands represent normal hair and are interspersed by abnormal dark bands where the medulla is expanded by air cavities that also spread into the cortex (Figure 8.8).

Monilethrix is a rare, autosomal dominantly inherited defect of the hair follicle characterized by keratosis pilaris, beaded hairs and fragile hair (Figure 8.9). This genetic defect leads to abnormal assembly of the keratin intermediate filaments resulting in the beading and fragility of the hair.

Figure 8.8
Appearance of pili annulati hair under the light microscope.

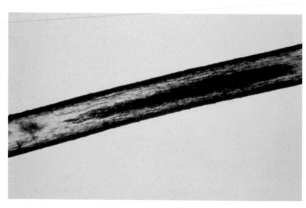

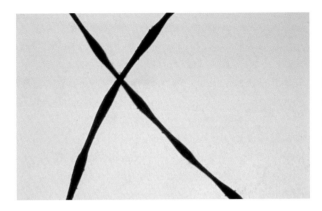

Figure 8.9
Microscopic appearance of the beaded hairs of monilethrix.

The beading may produce a slightly spangled appearance, but the dominant clinical presentation is with hair that fails to grow long due to fragility (Figure 8.10). Both beaded and non-beaded hairs are fragile. Beaded hairs may be hard to find and can represent less than 5% of scalp hairs.

The high but variable penetrance of the gene defect produces a wide spectrum of severity with some patients ostensibly normal and others unable to grow their hair more than a centimetre or two long. The clinical severity tends to remain constant throughout life.

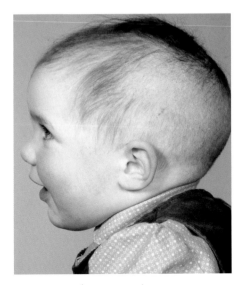

Figure 8.10
Clinical appearance of a child with monilethrix.

Netherton's syndrome. The hereditary association of a particular and distinctive ichthyosiform erythroderma called ichthyosis linearis circumflexa and fragile hair with invaginate nodes is known as Netherton's syndrome. Atopy is very common, occurring in up to 75% of cases. Failure to thrive in infancy is a potentially life-threatening complication and is due to the effects of the skin disease.

The most common hair change on light microscopy is the formation of trichorrhexis nodosa, however this change is non-specific and these nodes can be seen with hair weathering. Much less common are the invaginate nodes producing 'bamboo' hair (trichorrhexis invaginata); these are pathognomonic (Figure 8.11).

Trichothiodystrophy. The main barrier protecting hair from environmental injury is the hair cuticle. The strongest part of the cuticle is the sulphur-rich A layer. In trichothiodystrophy, a defect in the follicle prevents the high-sulphur proteins, such as cysteine, from migrating to the A layer, causing the band to fragment and rendering the hair susceptible to weathering.

For unknown reasons, when polarized the hairs have a banded appearance, reminiscent of a tiger tail (Figure 8.12). Although highly

(a)

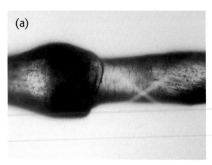

(b)

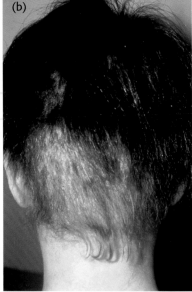

Figure 8.11 Netherton's syndrome:
(a) an invaginate (bamboo) node;
(b) clinical appearance of a child's hair.

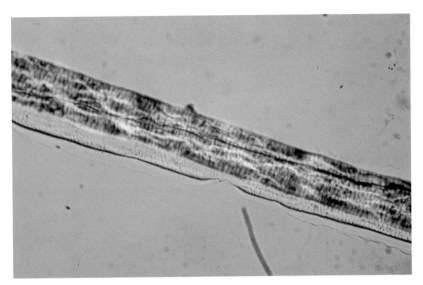

Figure 8.12 Microscopic appearance of hair in trichothiodystrophy.

suggestive of trichothiodystrophy, this sign is not pathognomonic and is seen in a number of other conditions. Demonstration of an absent A layer by transmission electron microscopy or sulphur deficiency in the hair by hydrolysis and two-dimensional electrophoresis and chromatography are required for diagnosis.

Clinically the patients may have hair fragility alone or it may be combined with ichthyosis, photosensitivity, decreased growth, impaired fertility or mental handicap (Table 8.4).

Loose anagen syndrome. Here, anchorage of growing anagen hairs to the follicle is impaired and these hairs can be easily and painlessly plucked from the follicle. As a result, most hairs do not remain *in situ* until completion of the anagen phase. This results in affected children having hair that does not grow long and that is of uneven lengths. Occasionally a schoolyard brawl will result in a clump of hair being pulled out to leave a bald patch. In addition, the hair is unruly and has an unusual sticky feel about it, though the cause of this is unknown.

Children between the ages of 2 and 7 years are most commonly affected. Their hair appears normal at birth, but becomes unruly, sticky and uneven at 2–3 years and remains so until it spontaneously becomes normal at

81

TABLE 8.4

Syndromes associated with trichothiodystrophy

	Photosensitivity	Intellectual impairment	Brittle, sulphur-deficient hair, often associated with brittle nails
Trichoschisis	–	–	+
Sabina's syndrome	–	–	+
BIDS syndrome	–	–	+
IBIDS or Tay's syndrome	–	+	+
PIBIDS syndrome	+	+	+
SIBIDS	–	+	+
ONMR syndrome	–	–	+
Marinesco–Sjögren's syndrome	–	–	+

BIDS, PIBIDS, IBIDS and SIBIDS are acronyms for individual features of the syndrome. B, brittle, sulphur-deficient hair often associated with brittle nails; I, intellectual impairment; D, decreased fertility; S, short stature; I, ichthyosis; P, photosensitivity; ONMR, onychotrichodysplasia, neutropenia, mental retardation

5–7 years. It is inherited as an autosomal dominant trait and it is common to find that apparently normal parents or older siblings also have the condition.

The characteristic light microscopy feature is that the hairs extracted by gentle traction are anagen hairs with mis-shapen bulbs, a crumpled proximal hair cuticle and without an inner root sheath.

Summary

An understanding of basic hair biology greatly enhances the assessment of the child with 'funny-looking' hair. In addition, approaching the problem according to the principal symptom, be it a disorder of hair volume or of the hair fibre itself, is more likely to lead to a diagnosis.

While the disorders discussed in this chapter are in general uncommon, it is important that they can be recognized for the purposes of diagnosing

Ichthyosis	Decreased fertility	Short stature	Neutropenia	Other abnormalities
–	–	–	–	
+	+	–	–	Ocular
+	+	+	–	Quadriplegia, fits
+	+	+	–	Dental, ocular and cardiac
+	+	+	+	Xeroderma pigmentosa
+	+	+	+	Osteosclerosis and cataracts
+	–	+	+	Recurrent infections
+	–	+	–	Neurological and dental

multisystem disorders, indicating a need for genetic counselling, for prognostic reasons and because hair disorders engender considerable anxiety among both parents and children.

CHAPTER 9

Future trends

Throughout the world, research is being undertaken into hair disorders, which is likely to affect their clinical management in the future. One of the most promising trends is the development of pharmaceutical agents, such as finasteride, that are specific antagonists or agonists of the biochemical pathways that affect hair growth. Such pathways not only include androgen metabolism, but also cytokines and growth factors such as vascular endothelial growth, transforming growth factor-β and insulin-like growth factor. The roles of these factors in hair growth and hair disorders are currently being investigated. Research into the role of the immune system in alopecia areata is proving to be particularly productive and should lead to new, more specific immunomodulatory treatments for this disorder.

The explosion in genetic research has included the genetic hair disorders. It is anticipated that the genes involved will be identified, which will provide further insights into the control of hair growth and structure. This could ultimately open the doorway for gene replacement as a treatment for these conditions.

Key references

Aram H. Treatment of female androgenetic alopecia with cimetidine. *Int J Dermatol* 1987;26:128–30.

Caputo R, Veraldi S. Erosive pustular dermatosis of the scalp. *J Am Acad Dermatol* 1993;28:96–8.

Dallob AL, Sadick NS, Unger O *et al.* The effect of finasteride, a 5α-reductase inhibitor on scalp skin testosterone and dihydrotestosterone concentration in patients with male pattern baldness. *J Clin Endocrinol Metab* 1994;79:703–6.

Dawber RPR. Aspects of treatment of scalp psoriasis. *J Dermatol Treat* 1989;1:103–5.

Dawber RD, ed. *Diseases of the Hair and Scalp*. 3rd edn. Oxford: Blackwell Science, 1997.

Burke BM, Cunliffe WJ. Oral spironolactone therapy for female patients with acne, hirsutism or androgenic alopecia. *Br J Dermatol* 1985;112:124–5.

Greer DL. Treatment of tinea capitis with itraconazole. *J Am Acad Dermatol* 1996; 35:637–40.

Gupta AK, Alexis ME, Raboobee N *et al.* Itraconazole pulse therapy is effective in the treatment of tinea capitis in children: an open multicentre study. *Br J Dermatol* 1997;137:251–4.

Jacobs JP, Szpunar CA, Warner ML. Use of topical minoxidil therapy for androgenetic alopecia in women. *Int J Dermatol* 1993;32:758–62.

Powell J, Dawber RPR, Gatter K. Folliculitis decalvans: the range of histological findings (communication). *Br Soc Dermatopathol*, January 1998.

Price VH. Topical minoxidil (3%) in extensive alopecia areata, including long term efficacy. *J Am Acad Dermatol* 1987;16:737–44.

Sawaya ME, Price VH. Different levels of 5α-reductase type I and II, aromatase, and androgen receptor in hair follicles of women and men with androgenetic alopecia. *J Invest Dermatol* 1997;109: 296–300.

Shaw JC. Antiandrogen therapy in dermatology. *Int J Dermatol* 1996; 35:770–8.

Solomon BA, Collins R, Sharma R *et al.* Fluconazole for the treatment of tinea capitis in children. *J Am Acad Dermatol* 1997;37:274–5.

Stenn KS, Messenger AG, Baden HP, eds. The molecular and structural biology of hair. *Ann NY Acad Sci* 1991;642.

Tosti A, De Padova MP, Minghetti G *et al.* Therapies versus placebo in the treatment of patchy alopecia areata. *J Am Acad Dermatol* 1986;15:209–10.

Van Neste D, Lachapelle JL, Antoine JL, eds. *Human Hair Growth and Alopecia Research*. Dordrecht: Kluwer Academic, 1989.

Index